DARE TO
Believe
FOR YOUR
Healing

Dare to Believe for Your Healing

VOICES OF HEALING WISDOM COMPILED BY

JULIA LOREN

WHITAKER
HOUSE

DARE TO BELIEVE FOR YOUR HEALING

ISBN: 978-1-62911-162-9
eBook ISBN: 978-1-62911-163-6

© 2014 by Julia Loren

Whitaker House
1030 Hunt Valley Circle
New Kensington, PA 15068
www.whitakerhouse.com

Library of Congress Cataloging-in-Publication Data (Pending)

This book has been printed digitally and produced in a standard specification in order to ensure its continuing availability.

CONTENTS

"God is kind, preferring that His children be well rather than sick."

"Jesus was always kind and considerate in praying for the sick and showing love and affection. He never scolded anyone for his condition."

"Divine healing is neither automatic nor dependent on our right actions. Healing is not a formula, nor does it come from man-made methods. We need to remember healing is a gift from God rooted in deep relationship with the power of His Spirit."

"Healing is always God's desire."

—John Wimber

PREFACE

I pray that you will be blessed by this compilation of writings from Christians of strong faith from both the past and present who collectively show us that God still delights in manifesting supernatural healing today. At the end of each excerpt, you will find a section called "Journey into Word & Spirit." This segment provides questions for you to examine and action steps/points of obedience for you to follow that will lead you to experience healing in your own life. As you *Dare to Believe for Your Healing,* put your faith into practice immediately and watch what God will do!

INTRODUCTION

Yesterday

It was late in the day, and I was too tired to continue skiing, but I ignored the warning of my better judgment—as well as the prompting of the Holy Spirit—to ride the gondola back down to the bottom of the hill. Instead, I decided to go for one last run.

That wasn't the only time I'd ignored the Holy Spirit in recent days. I'd had two choices for how to spend this weekend—visiting Christian friends outside London, where I would enjoy the fellowship of like-minded believers, or skiing with colleagues in Austria. It had long been a dream of mine to ski the Alps, and I'd thought this would likely be my only opportunity, so I'd seized the day. But, suddenly, the day "seized" me. It turned out to be "one last run," indeed! I had a spectacular wipeout on the mountain—sliding, skidding, and rolling probably a hundred feet down a steep, icy run. Along the way, I heard an odd popping sound in my knee and thought, *That can't be good.*

When I finally came to a halt, my head was facing down the mountain, and my skis were above my head. I flipped myself around so that my legs would lie below my head, and then I stood, only to feel my left knee buckle. I was forced to sit back down, because I was not able to put any weight on my knee. The evening darkness was descending quickly in that little, out-of-the-way run, and the ski patrol was nowhere to be found. One of my colleagues snowboarded over and asked if I was hurt. I said yes. In total sincerity, knowing that, in that place, being rescued was not possible, he gazed at me with the most compassionate eyes and said, "Suck it up. You must try."

So, I had no choice but to ski all the way down the mountain—a twenty-minute run under normal circumstances. I realized that I could put weight on my leg only if I skied straight ahead—something you don't do on a steep, bumpy slope. I was not able to turn to the right without my leg buckling, but I could turn to the left if I shifted all my weight onto my right leg.

So, with tears in my eyes, I pointed my skis down the slope and then turned left, maneuvering my weight appropriately, and slowly skied sideways down the mountain. But the "little bumps," or moguls, on the run obstructed my path. I started praying in earnest, "Please, God, help me get down this mountain." And I repeated the verse *"I can do all things through Christ who strengthens me"* (Philippians 4:13 NKJV). And strength flowed in.

I have to ski. In ten minutes, the mountain will be dark, I told myself. I was barely able to see the run in front of me. I fell again, groaning with the exertion of getting up, and then again as I tried to ski on one leg. Repeating this chain of events, I managed to ski the rest of the way down on one leg without falling—stopping every twenty feet or so for a few seconds' rest. Then, I slowly and cautiously limped to the bus, afraid of the damage—and angry at myself.

Day 1

I sit alone in an Austrian hotel room with my knee swollen and my leg propped up as I finish writing this manuscript. My colleagues are skiing the sunny slopes of the Austrian Alps without me. And two important questions are flying through my mind: *Will God heal me as He heals others?* and—oddly enough—*Do I want to be healed?*

I contemplate the end of my "skiing career" and hobble about the hotel room. I have no idea of the extent of the damage to my knee from the previous day's wipeout. I haven't yet seen a doctor, so I am without crutches, braces, or the ability to put weight on my leg, especially when I turn. I still have muscle spasms in my good leg from the strain of the last run.

I start e-mailing friends to pass the time. "Probably a torn meniscus," a friend wrote back. "Probably a bad sprain," another e-mailed with a more hopeful diagnosis. I am icing my knee, praying, and contemplating the repercussions of going against my better judgment. I am convinced that I should have taken the route of a more faith-building, kingdom-expanding time of fellowship rather than the route of skiing the Alps, which had effectively ended on that body-demolishing, icy slope. I am convicted that I am, once again, out of God's will and in my own will.

As I review this book and recall so many stories of faith, and as I read Scriptures that reveal the compassionate love of God, I wonder, *Will God heal my knee, or will He let me experience the consequences of my own sin of stepping out of His will? Will He heal me despite my own folly?*

I remember reading Guillermo Maldonado's book *The Kingdom of Power: How to Demonstrate It Here and Now*, in which he wrote, "We may have faith to believe and to declare a manifestation from the eternal realm, but if we are not right with God in any area of our lives, our faith can be nullified." I realize that my conscience has been condemning me and blocking me from receiving healing, and I earnestly repent. But I wonder if I have just said some words to get something from God—like the miracle of instant healing.

Then I hear the voice of the Lord speak to my heart: *Why wouldn't I heal you? Everyone has sinned and fallen short of My glory. But your sin was paid for on the cross. You have brought the matter before Me and repented, and you feel contrite about it. And whoever comes to Me, I will not send away. You have asked for forgiveness, and My blood covers you. You can punish yourself by accepting the pain and swollenness of your leg, going to a doctor for a diagnosis, and hobbling about as long as you wish. Or, you can accept My healing, for I am the One who forgives ALL your sin and heals ALL your diseases.* (See Psalm 103:3.)

Randy Clark said, "Healing is grace based." Grace covers me. It is something I cannot earn. It is God's gift. His grace forgives. His grace heals. He loves both you and me.

Andrew Murray wrote, "Happy is he who comes to understand that it is the will of God to heal, to manifest the power of Jesus, and to reveal to us His fatherly love. It is also His will that we exercise and confirm our faith, to make us prove the power of redemption in the body as well as in the soul." The Father loves me. Why wouldn't He heal my body? After all, He has saved—and is saving—my soul.

And so I respond in faith. There is no feeling of His presence, no goose bumps of the gift of faith flooding into me. But I take Him at His Word, right here and right now. I pray, "Lord, I accept Your gift of healing. Release Your healing presence to me. Please, Abba, You who are good, kind, and miraculous, You who say that healing is the 'children's bread,' You who are full of compassion, Jehovah-Rapha, come. Heal me. I welcome You here."

I take authority over my body and command the swelling to go down, the cartilage to be restored, and the muscles to regain strength, releasing the healing power of Christ into my leg. I wait on the Lord, giving Him thanks and praise.

I turn on some music and begin to worship, and I feel the pain leave and the swelling subside within the hour. A measure of healing has come, and I am totally excited!

Day 2

I haven't been praying for a miracle or an instantaneous cure, but rather for healing—which is often progressive. My healing is still in progress, but it is apparent that I should now seek medical attention. So, two days after the "big crash," one of my colleagues drives me back to Germany, where I have been doing some consulting work. I limp into a local hospital. Initially, the orthopedic physician diagnoses me with a torn medial collateral ligament (MCL), gives me a soft cast, and says I should stay off my feet for a week before seeing if the leg will support my weight. Four to six weeks of recovery should be sufficient, he assures me—if there are no other undetected damages. However, an MRI reveals a completely torn anterior cruciate ligament (ACL), with meniscus damage and hip strain.

I return to my hotel room, prop up my leg on the couch, and continue working on the introduction to this book. I feel that I am now faced with another dilemma, in which I have three choices: Ask the Lord for an instant miracle, continue to ask the Lord to heal me, or use this injury as my ticket home, so that I can spend the Christmas holidays in the USA rather than remain in Germany for another five weeks. I have faith for a miracle. I have faith that God will heal me—with or without someone else praying for me. But do I really want Him to?

I imagine the "benefits" of being injured and somewhat incapacitated. I can have people wait on me. I can wallow in front of the television all day, eating chocolate, if I want to. No one will expect much from me. It sounds pretty good—if only I wasn't in pain. *I wouldn't mind sitting at home in front of my fireplace right now*, I think, *planning Christmas with friends and family.* But I can't let myself walk away from a work assignment just because I am homesick. I can, however, tell my supervisor about my medical condition and be sent home...unless God miraculously heals my knee and "wrecks" that plan.

On a less superficial level, I recognize some positive outcomes of my being injured. Filled with new compassion for the frail and ill, I begin to view the elderly in a new way. The old woman I see crossing the street is moving exceedingly slow for a reason—not to aggravate drivers who wait for her to cross, but because she has limited mobility and is perhaps in pain. I feel more tenderness toward my elderly mother, who has courageously traveled to many doctors' appointments and surgeries in recent years without anyone's support or assistance. It was unpleasant for me, at my age, to have to go to the hospital, but it must be frightening for her at her age. So, newfound compassion is a benefit of my immobility. I will keep that renewed perspective long after I am healed.

But my question is still this: Do I want God to heal me, or do I want the advantages of remaining unhealed for a while (going home for the holidays and paying my mortgage with medical and financial benefits)? Granted, a torn MCL is a common injury, and I was assured it would heal on its own, eventually. It was not life threatening—just inconvenient. But the principles of healing still applied to it.

I have settled my first question, *Will God heal me...?* I know He forgives all my sins and heals all my diseases. But I have yet to decide if I *want* to be healed—a condition that would call me to give up the "perks" of affliction.

If you are battling an injury or an illness, you may have to settle some questions, too. You may need to prepare yourself to receive your healing. I will leave the outcome of my own experience open-ended so that you can personally explore the issues of healing presented in this book.

Do You Believe in Healing?

Are you convinced that Jesus will heal you or extend His miraculous touch on your behalf? Do you *want* to be healed?

If you are facing a terminal diagnosis, that second question is even more profound for you than it is for those who are dealing with chronic or short-term illnesses. Do you want to be healed, or do you want to go home to be with the Lord? I remember hearing a story about my late friend Jill Austin, who heard the Lord speak to her heart as she squirmed in painful agony on her hospital bed. She said she was faced with the choice of going home to be with the Lord or continuing to live here on earth. She chose to be with her heavenly Father; and, soon after making that conscious decision, she passed.

You may need to ask yourself whether God is calling you home. If so, your prayers (and the prayers of others) should be directed to Him accordingly. I have heard many stories of people who realized it was time for them to move on, and who died well. They passed quickly, easily—falling asleep and waking up in the arms of heaven's embrace.

However, if you are wrestling with issues of faith concerning healing, and if you want to be healed, read on. The chapters in this book were written by pioneers of the healing movement—those with gifts of healings and miracles—and gifted teachers. Their writings will strengthen your faith and prepare you to receive healing. God will heal you. His promises are *yes* and *amen*. (See 2 Corinthians 1:20.) Healing is for you—today.

Experience God's Grace

Enter into God's grace as you read this book. If you find that your heart leaps or your head tingles when you come across a particular Scripture, teaching, or phrase, that sensation is the Holy Spirit saying, "Pay attention! This is a promise for you to hold on to, an access point though which you can enter into, and receive, heaven's healing." Start praying that promise. Be encouraged.

Dare to believe.
God has not forgotten you.
He is closer to you than your own heart.
His love and compassion are here, now, for you.

May you be blessed, may your faith rise to new heights, and may you be healed before you finish reading this book.

LAYING HOLD OF HOPE BEYOND REASON

Julia Loren

1

LAYING HOLD OF HOPE
BEYOND REASON

Julia Loren

"The Lord will sustain him on his sickbed
and restore him from his bed of illness."
—Psalm 41:3 (NIV)

Those who receive healing always grab hold of a measure of faith when a particular Scripture leaps off the page and into their hearts, or in a moment when the Holy Spirit speaks directly to their hearts in prayer, or by way of someone else's faith, one who has received a word of knowledge or inspiration from the Holy Spirit. Faith is key to receiving healing. Faith for healing arises when you hold onto either your own faith or another person's faith. Those who receive healing almost always first receive a gift of faith, which the current of heaven rides upon to wash away pain and disease.

Faith is the container of "hope beyond reason"—the expectation of unseen things coming to pass. Faith is ignited in a community that welcomes the presence of the Lord. Faith receives the power of God, who loves you.

The following thoughts on faith and hope are from my book When God Says Yes.

When I see extraordinary miracles in the lives of the people I meet, I hear a common theme of events that contributed to their healing. First, they received bad news. Then they received personal, specific words from the Lord that contradicted the death sentence and infused them with hope. And throughout the long ordeal that tested their faith, others helped them hold onto a hope beyond reason.

The following stories are about two very different individuals who entered into a hope beyond reason, felt the support of a loving community, and received a miraculous healing. One is an American pastor who was healed of leukemia. The other is an African woman living in Rome, Italy, who was healed of acute depression and psychotic episodes that she was prone to under the weight of grief. I include their stories because cancer and depression claim more lives than we care to admit. The testimonies of their healings speak to all those who have physical or mental illness that seems incurable. Nothing is incurable for Jesus. He who created us can uncreate disease and re-create health, giving us all that we need for life. Our Creator is the God of the miraculous.

Dave Hess is one of the most unassuming, soft-spoken, humble men I have ever met. Pastor of a large church in Pennsylvania, he and his family walked down a long road of debilitating illness and recovery several years ago. I sobbed my way through his book *Hope Beyond Reason*, which tells the story of his ordeal. I cried not out of sadness. Yes, the book detailed a lot of grief and pain I cannot imagine enduring, but it was far from sad. Rather, I cried because of the beauty this book revealed about faith, hope, and love. Dave's faith, as he held onto the promises of God, revealed an amazing desire to live. His family and the community of his church constantly held out hope and interceded night and day for several months. Their intercessions created an atmosphere of faith that not only broke through for Dave's healing, but released a breakthrough ministry of healing throughout the church.

What brought tears to my eyes most often was the beautiful love story he wove through his book. The love between husband and wife, father and children, pastor and church, God and man splashed out from the pages and washed over me as I read. The brief synopsis of his story that I include here gives but a glimpse into how one man held onto a handful of promises and received the miraculous provision of healing.

Immediately after Dave Hess was given the news that he had advanced leukemia and needed to enter the hospital immediately, Dave heard the Lord give him a promise that implied he would not die, but would live. As he drove home to tell his family about the diagnosis the doctor had given him, he sensed the Lord speaking words of hope out of Hosea chapter 2. Here is Dave's story:

I will allure her, bring her into the wilderness, and speak kindly to her. Then I will give her her vineyards from there, and the valley of Achor as a door of hope. And she will sing there as in the days of her youth.

(Hosea 2:14–15 NASB)

In this valley of tears, that same Lord was opening a door of hope for me.

As I turned the corner of our street and drove toward the house, I noticed a number of cars in our driveway. Opening the door from the garage, I was welcomed by a kitchen filled with family and friends. Waves of love broke over me as I walked through the door. My parents-in-law were there, along with my sister-in-law Robin. Our friend Karna and our youth pastor Tom had also rallied to the call. Upon hearing a vague report that something might be wrong, they had dropped everything to stand with us in prayer. A cavalcade of phone calls was already alerting others to pray. Within a few short hours, a small army was sounding the battle cry.

Questioning looks encircled the room. I wanted to give all of them answers. But glimpsing at the faces of Sheri and the children, I drew them aside to tell them first.

Crouching to look at them eye-to-eye, I heard myself say, "Daddy has cancer. But Jesus has Daddy."

Together we melted into one big hug, mixed with tears. We felt hands on our heads and shoulders as those we love lifted us up to the One who loves. We embraced one another, and we sensed His embrace.

A few days later, reflecting on this moment, I would write these words in my journal:

> What a whirlwind this has been. Yet, what a wonderful "eye" in this storm. Promises abound in this time. Scriptures and personal words keep coming to me with the constant and sweet reminding of the Holy Spirit. There *is* a door of Hope in this valley of troubling! I am watching as the Lord wars against my demonic enemies (Nahum 1:2–6). At the same time, He is fortifying me with His peace, His faith, and His presence (Nahum 1:7–10). Keep rejoicing!

Habakkuk 3:19 in the *Amplified Bible* says:

The Lord God is my strength, my personal bravery, and my invincible army...and will make me to walk [not to stand still in terror, but to walk] and make [spiritual] progress upon my high places [of trouble, suffering, or responsibility].

That night I slept like a child, safe in the arms of my Father. He is my strength. He is my personal bravery. He is my invincible army. I will not stand still in terror. Instead, I will make spiritual progress upon my high places of trouble. These words ran through my mind and out of my mouth.

For the next six months, Dave lived mostly in the hospital as he battled the cancer. Twice, the doctors said he had only hours to live. Twice, Dave stepped away from death and back into life. During his weakest moments of faith, God released others with the right word to restore his hope beyond reason. Dave tells of one such meeting:

> One day a thirteen-year-old girl named Mary stepped into our lives. She had urged her mother to bring her to the hospital to see us, saying she had something she needed to tell us. Mary had been diagnosed with ovarian cancer earlier that year. A large tumor had been removed, yet doctors were uncertain about her chances for a full recovery. One day while reading her Bible, Mary came across this verse in Psalms:

I will not die but live, and will proclaim what the LORD *has done* (Psalm 118:17).

It spoke hope to her in her valley of trouble. Here she stood beside my bed, cancer-free. The tumor was gone and Mary's life had been restored. She lived, and she was telling me what the Lord had done. Mary held out a handwritten note card with Psalm 118:17 printed on it. "I hung this by my bed when I was in the hospital," she said with a sparkle in her eyes. "It gave me hope. I want you to have hope, too. You're not going to die. You're going to live, too!"

Then she prayed for us. Her words were pure expressions of trust, voiced to a God she had found to be trustworthy.

With a confident smile, Mary looked at me and said once more, "You will not die. You will live. And you will tell everyone what the Lord has done."

After Mary and her mother left the room, Sheri opened the mail. Included in all the expressions of support were *five* cards with Psalm 118:17 written in them. The Lord's faithful promises were calling us to a deeper place of trust! "I will not die but live, and will proclaim what the Lord has done."

Together we laughed. It was not the laughter of a humorous diversion. Rather it was a confident laughter, given to us as a gift from the Lord, born out of the relief that comes from knowing we can trust Him. He was showering us with reminders of His strong presence to sustain us. The Bible frequently says the Lord brings confirmation through two or three witnesses. We had received a word confirmed by six witnesses! I guess we needed all of them.

While Dave battled in the hospital, his church battled on the home front. It has been said that nothing happens unless we pray; and that God moves mountains in response to prayers of faith. But I also believe that there is a hidden truth in the psalmist's words in Psalm 133:1–3, that where brethren dwell together in unity—there the oil runs freely down the faces of the prayer warriors, cascading joyfully out the door like the swollen streams of winter's melting snowpack, spilling over onto the streets, and running into the byways and hospitals and even to nations far beyond the walls of any church building. Dave relates how his congregation stepped into a unity of spirit that released both the prophetic and healing anointing oil in their midst:

> On her way home that evening, Sheri noticed that the lights were on at the church and the parking lot was filled with cars. She knew of no scheduled meeting, so she pulled in, curious to see what was going on. As she entered the sanctuary, she was amazed to see hundreds of people engaged in prayer.
>
> At the front of the church was our dear friend Dawn Sweigart leading the charge. Dawn had surrendered her life to Jesus just a few years prior. She had come to Him with a wide-open heart that seemed to blossom overnight. She was a leader, an influencer, a motivator and a budding prophet. She heard the voice of the Lord and sensed His heartbeat in an extremely unique way. She expressed it in an equally distinctive way. We deeply loved her.
>
> Just moments after learning the news of my illness, she rallied hundreds of people from our church and our region to pray. As a young follower of Jesus, Dawn had taken hold of His promises with tenacity. If He said He would do miracles, then He would do miracles! If He said we would do greater works than He did (John 14:12), then we will do greater works than He did! Her heart throbbed with the conviction that He will make His promises a reality in our day!
>
> Dawn had organized round-the-clock prayer for us. People volunteered to pray for an hour each week, collectively covering all 168 hours of the week. Local pastors and their congregations joined us, and various prayer gatherings spontaneously sprang up in response to the needs of the moment and the Holy Spirit's leading. This is what Jesus said His Church would look like. More than buildings, organizations, politics or programs, He builds His Church with people. He draws those who are being rescued and restored, as well as those now devoting their lives to rescuing and restoring others.
>
> There is nothing more beautiful on the planet than when followers of Jesus act like Jesus. On the other hand, there is nothing more

grievous than when believers in Jesus don't even resemble Him. Some like to throw stones at the Church in moments like these, seeing her as detestable. Out of touch. Past her prime. But as author Fawn Parish quips, "The Church is like Noah's ark. It stinks but it's the only thing afloat." She goes on to say, "When we criticize the Church, we are criticizing something Jesus adores and spilled His blood for. It is His own precious possession."

Night after night these prayer warriors met. Often sharing in communion, they would declare the power of Jesus' victory over sin, sickness, death and all of the forces of hell. They spent hours together worshiping, encouraging one another and interceding.

But they were not just praying for me. They were asking the Lord to touch every life in our region and beyond!

Faith and fervency erupted in people's hearts throughout the congregation. Many who did not see themselves as prayer warriors boldly enlisted in this holy war. It was an all-out fight for the hearts and lives of those in our territory. Mindful of the eternal consequences, we continue to pray for every orphaned heart to know and receive the love of their Father through His amazing Son, Jesus!

What could have intimidated us ignited us.

Fresh doors of hope were being opened in this valley of trouble.

Just when it seemed that the leukemia was in remission, the medical treatments caused Dave's body to react in such a way that Dave almost died—for a second time. Once again, Dave and Sheri stood and declared the promises of God, and once again, Dave stepped away from the door of death and back to the door of hope. But they still had a ways to go through the valley of trouble.

One day, Dave's appendix burst, and due to his weakened condition, doctors determined that they could not operate. They told Sheri that Dave will surely die. However, Dave had been given other promises, divine encounters with prayer, and knew that he would not die. At one point, healing evangelist Randy Clark came to his hospital and prayed an unusual prayer—not just for healing of the leukemia, but for the healing of his abdominal area. At the time, it seemed unusual. But when Dave's appendix burst, Randy's prayer became another promise to hold onto.

The doctors told Sheri that no one lived longer than a couple of horrendously painful days with a burst appendix. They could not operate due to Dave's weakened condition and decided to send him home with hospice care to die in the company of his family. But his family and friends continued to hold onto the promises of healing, and Dave continued to survive:

Finally, after six weeks, my blood levels were restored. With white cells, red cells and platelets in healthy balance, I met with the surgeon to prepare for surgery.

"I've looked over your charts," he said. "You've had a ruptured appendix inside you for over six weeks. I'm going to do an exploratory procedure on you because I'm not sure what we will find. The poison that is secreted from a burst appendix is highly toxic. We need to see what damage has been done to your internal organs."

Grateful to be alive, I underwent surgery the next morning. As I nodded off, counting backwards at the direction of the anesthetist, I remembered Jesus' promise to me. *You are a shield around me*, I said to Him as I drifted off into an anesthetic fog.

Later in the recovery room, the surgeon greeted Sheri and me. His first words to us were exclamations of amazement: "I've never seen anything like this!" Holding up four snapshots, he said, "Look at these pictures!"

They were pictures of my insides. In 5x7 glossy prints. Suitable for framing.

"Here," he said, pointing at one of the photos, "is your appendix, or what is left of it. Amazingly, it is encased inside a tent-like structure that completely encompasses your appendix! Did you ever have an operation in this part of your body?" he asked.

"Not that I remember," I responded. "Why do you ask?"

"Because this tent is composed of adhesions. It's the strongest type of scar tissue your body can manufacture. This kind of scar tissue only appears after someone has had surgery! It appears to have been in place before your appendix ruptured. All of the poison was contained inside it," he said, while making a circular gesture on the photo. "Not a drop of poison escaped this tent. Your entire internal system is as healthy as that of a twenty year old!" *What a compliment!* I thought.

Bewildered, relieved, grateful and amazed, I asked him, "What did this tent of adhesions look like?"

"That's the funniest thing," he said curiously. "It looked like a group of shields that had been sewn together!"

Just as He promised, so He had done. The Lord had miraculously created a miracle pouch. A tent of shields. Grabbing my Bible, I opened once again to the passage containing His timely word to us. I marvel at it to this day.

> *Many are saying of me, "God will not deliver him." But you are a shield around me, O LORD (Psalm 3:2–3).*

Just as God shielded Dave from death, God covers us all with His shield of salvation. Many say of those with fatal illness that God will not deliver them. Even those who struggle with chronic mental illness are deemed incurable by man or by God. Yet, holding onto the promises of God—despite evidence to the contrary—increases faith. When others draw near in love (rather than in unbelief), miracles happen. Community becomes the container of faith that holds us and shields us from the enemy's schemes. Community releases the love that empowers us to continue to hold onto hope beyond reason. Dave's family joined forces with a church community that did not waver in unbelief. And Dave was completely healed. More than ten years later, Dave remains healthy, without a trace of cancer.

While God can move and does move in response to our faith alone, the healing power seems most quickly released when a community of believers stands with the one in need.

Community—the Container of Hope

I first noticed this amplified healing response of community while speaking at a women's retreat in Rome, Italy, some years ago. When I came in contact with another woman who was in desperate need of healing, I noticed that the miracle she received came as a result of a community drawing her into their circle of love and interceding for her day and night. This kind of love seems rare in our western culture. Perhaps that is why God modeled it for me in the African community long before I was able to see it modeled through the Pennsylvania church in Dave Hess's story.

Elsie shuffled into the retreat, accompanied by two other African women, her eyes obviously deadened by a powerful antipsychotic. She was suicidal. Her whole world shattered when her boyfriend abandoned her and state child protection authorities took her infant daughter away until she could regain her sanity. Her African "sisters" brought her to this retreat held at an oceanside community near Rome, Italy, in hopes that God would touch her and make her whole.

Only they knew what had really happened to Elsie in her past. I could only guess what leads an African woman to leave her country, family, and friends for a foreign land to earn enough money to send home and sustain, perhaps, the whole village. Poverty, sexual abuse, war, and the threat of AIDS probably all contributed to her arrival in Italy, where she worked as a domestic employee in a land prejudiced against her. The stress of moving to another country is enough to unsettle anyone. Add a string of traumas occurring both before and after the move, and that pressure would challenge the coping ability of even the toughest individual. It was no surprise that Elsie's ability to cope had shattered into a million pieces.

After her breakdown, doctors on a hospital mental ward told her she was suffering from major depression with psychotic features. They stabilized her with heavy doses of medication and, several weeks later, said she could go home. Once Elsie was released from the hospital, her African friends, her sisters, took her in, watched over her, prayed for her, and drew her nearer to the fires of God's love.

After several months of watching and praying over her night and day, they brought her with them to this retreat on the outskirts of Rome, by the sea, where the pastors of a large Assemblies of God church in Rome had invited me to speak....It was here in Italy that I met Elsie and stood in awe of God, watching His presence move powerfully, healing her and many other women from depression and anxiety during the retreat and in the weeks following. It was here that I came to understand the demonic component of depression and despair and watched God shatter the "spirit of despair" in the lives of many, freeing them to dance in the fullness of joy.

Elsie was one of the first to be healed. She stood for prayer, and as I made my way down the line, she stared straight ahead as if completely unaware of what was happening. Either that or she was scared to death. I didn't even know if she spoke English, but I noticed that no one translated for her into either an African or Italian language. I paused before her, raised my hand to her forehead, and before I could utter a word, she crumbled to the floor. During both the evening and morning sessions, she stood for prayer and immediately fell into a deeper encounter with the presence of God. Each time I walked on, wondering what she felt, wondering if she just fell down out of preconditioned expectation. I felt nothing. Jet lag diminished the sense of God's presence, and I just went through the motions of speaking and praying, confident that the women were receiving something of God's power and presence and prophetic words. What I felt was of no consequence. What they felt was!

The afternoon session was devoted initially to testimonies of what God was doing in individual lives so far. Two women shared freely. Then Elsie abruptly shuffled up to me. Many in the audience stiffened, afraid that she would disrupt the meeting with insane chatter. As I held the microphone for her, she testified in fairly clear English the story of her fall into sin, the trauma of losing her baby to the state, her salvation, and her sense of God's presence healing her that weekend. Her African sisters sat listening, wiping tears from their eyes. For indeed, a change had come over Elsie—her eyes were clearer, and her speech, though tainted by medication, showed clarity of thought and a logical flow of content as she told her saga.

Her descent into depression originated in loneliness that led her into a relationship with a man who used her sexually—with no thought of love or commitment. As a result, she became pregnant. And when she gave birth, the authorities took away her child. It sounds similar to what David and Bathsheba experienced in 2 Samuel 11–12. The problems of illicit sex, unre-solved relationship issues, and unrepentant affairs always open the soul to the spirit of despair. However, God was out to destroy the works of the enemy and redeem Elsie's life from the pit, despite her having to walk through the consequences of her choices.

I stood beside Elsie and noticed many Europeans squirm in their seats while she spoke. When she finished, I simply prayed, "Father, we hear her story as a confession of how she has sinned and how You are redeeming her. Now we as representatives of the Church forgive her, and You forgive her. Release her into the complete healing You have for her. Destroy the work of the evil one that seeks to rob her of the fullness of life and joy and peace."

At that, her eyes rolled back in her head until all I could see was solid white. Rustling in the seats drew my attention, and I nodded at a couple of her sisters to come up. They took her to a corner of the room and quietly delivered her of the unclean spirit that had attached itself to her during this traumatic phase of grief and loss.

On the following Wednesday night, I spoke at a large meeting in Rome and saw Elsie waiting at the door.

"Elsie! What has happened? You look so full of joy!"

"Oh, Julia," she replied, "I got very sick when I left the retreat and had to go to hospital. The doctor told me that they had to get me off all medication quickly. I am healed."

Indeed, she was.

A year later, the Italian authorities refused to release her child to her custody. She fell into a depression for a short while. However, she had spent the year growing in her relationship with God and living in community with people who loved and cared for her, draping the garments of salvation around her shoulders on a daily basis. Her depression lifted quickly as she realized that *"hope deferred makes the heart sick"* (Proverbs 13:12 NKJV), and she sought Jesus for healing. She walked through this period without medication, nor did she require hospitalization. She is fine today, coping without falling into depression...despite her challenging circumstances.

Dave Hess, Elsie, and many others have received healing in the company of others. It is the nature of God to enable the body to "build itself up in love." When people come together, God is present in their midst. The enemy knows this, and so he moves in like a lion targeting its prey to cut it off from the rest of the herd so he can close in and kill.

Each one in these stories listened for the promise of the Lord specific to their need and declared it over themselves—or others declared it over them in intercession. Faith stirred in someone's life, and God rushed in to meet it, for God is attracted more to faith than to unbelief.

God Will Heal All of Your Diseases

Jesus doesn't want the evil one to succeed in destroying you. He wants to destroy the enemy's power over you that manifests in your life as depression and anxiety. His love for you leads you to understand that you can run to Jesus rather than hide in isolation. His love for you is even now breaking off the spirit of despair that so often accompanies long-term illness.

> Bless the LORD, O my soul, and forget none of His benefits; who pardons all your iniquities; who heals all your diseases; who redeems your life from the pit; who crowns you with lovingkindness and compassion; who satisfies your years with good things, so that your youth is renewed like the eagle. (Psalm 103:2–5 NASB)

According to this passage in Psalms 103, He will heal all your diseases, redeem your life from the pit of depression and anxiety, release an overwhelming sense of His love and kindness toward you, and increase your understanding of His compassion. It is part of the package called salvation.

God's Word, the Bible, is full of promises that speak of entering into the fullness of salvation. Every time I read it, God seems to make the words come alive. God speaks personally to me—through His Word and through the Word quickened to my spirit. When you are walking through the valley of trouble, reading the Word will reveal the door of hope. It will also break through any self-defeating thoughts that seek to hinder your healing and rob your joy.

Lest you think that miracles of healing are only for special people, let me assure you that you, too, are special. Made in the image of God, you are a child of God. His delight is in you. He does not will that anyone should suffer or be ill. If you doubt that, listen to what Dave Hess has to say about the lessons he learned in the midst of his illness.

Somewhere along the line, we have been lied to. We were told that God sends us sickness to teach us a lesson. At the same time, we were told He doesn't do miracles anymore, that He somehow "got it out of His system" when Jesus walked the earth. In fact, this lie went so far as to say if someone claims to have experienced a miracle, Satan probably had something to do with it.

I pondered this for a moment.

God gives us diseases? And Satan works miracles?

What a clever con!

This miracle we were experiencing was not a rare occurrence. In fact, what we call miracles, He calls normal. When Jesus said signs and wonders would follow those who believe Him, He did not use the word *occasionally*. And I was not getting special treatment simply because I was a pastor. He promises to give good gifts to all His children. He doesn't show partiality. He is not a shifty carnival worker who occasionally lets someone win in order to keep the rest of the customers at the counter. Though we have tried to change Him, He has not changed. He is still the God of miracles. He is still the One with Whom nothing is impossible. Nothing is too hard for Him! We can trust Him. We can hope in Him. Not because we are gullible, but because He is believable!

Dave and Elsie received specific promises from the Lord for healing. The promises they held onto are for you, too.

Journey into Word & Spirit

1. What Scripture from this chapter stood out to you? Write it down as a reminder of the promise that God has given specifically to you.

2. Is there a person in your life who is standing with you in prayer? Or, do you know of a person who will stand with you in prayer if requested? Why not ask him or her to do so?

3. Has there been a specific moment on your journey toward health and healing when God has intervened and given you hope? What happened? Be specific.

Chapter excerpted from Julia Loren, *When God Says Yes: His Promise and Provision When You Need It Most* (Grand Rapids: MI: Chosen Books, a division of Baker Publishing Group, 2010), 80–94. Used by permission. The portion in italics at the beginning was added by the writer for this publication.

About the Author

Julia Loren is a prolific writer who has authored more than a dozen books, as well as many poems and short stories. She earned a bachelor of arts degree in journalism from the University of Washington and a master's degree in counseling and psychology from Seattle Pacific University. Since her early professional days as a journalist, she has channeled her skills into helping people to realize their gifts and to walk in their God-given destinies.

Julia is a sought-after speaker at community events and churches, and she conducts writing workshops throughout the year. She resides north of Seattle, Washington, and takes frequent trips to the sunny shores of California.

For more information on Julia Loren, visit www.bluemothmedia.com and www.amazon.com/author/julialoren.

THE PURPOSE OF
THE TESTIMONY

Bill Johnson

2

THE PURPOSE OF THE TESTIMONY

Bill Johnson

*"Your testimonies I have taken as a heritage forever,
for they are the rejoicing of my heart."*
—Psalm 119:111 (NKJV)

When we hear testimonies of what God has done, they are not just stories to applaud; they are prophecies to receive. Revelation 19:10 reads, *"The testimony of Jesus is the spirit of prophecy."* Behind every testimony of victory, healing, salvation, and restoration is a power and grace contained in that prophetic declaration for God to do it again in your life, family, and city. The testimony is the spoken or written record of God's works that reveal His nature and demonstrate His covenant with man. God is using the record of His supernatural works to build a reference point upon which His Kingdom is advancing. When we report stories about heaven breaking into earth, each is a reminder of God's covenant with us. It prophesies the nature of God revealing His intention, not just for an individual or a one-time event, but to create a ripple effect where power and grace is released on the body of Christ to receive the breakthrough prophesied every time the testimony is declared. God is looking for agreement on earth—declarations that invite His invasion.

The power of speaking out the testimony of God's works creates an atmosphere of faith that expands your world that you influence. It shapes your prayer life, how you see God, and what you declare, so that you look at impossibilities from the victorious perspective of heaven. When you read these stories, you will meet the Jesus who heals, who calls forth people into their destinies, and who demonstrates His love and power through encounter.

Each story invites the reader into a lifestyle of encountering the same God.... As we become keepers of our own testimony, we make our experience available for others. [Testimonies of healing] are your inheritance to receive as prophetic promises for God to do it again in your own life, with your family, with your friends, within your city.

Revelation 12:11 states that they overcame him [Satan] by the blood of the lamb and the power of the testimony. The blood of the Lamb is what bought the victory. The word of the testimony releases the power. The power is released when you declare it. The person with the experience is never at the mercy of the person with the argument.

Journey into Word & Spirit

1. Have you ever heard or read a testimony of healing of a condition that is similar to yours? Write it down as a prophetic promise that God is giving specifically to you.

2. Write out a declaration that the Lord will heal you and then speak it out loud.

3. Recall and write down a testimony of the Lord ministering in your life and touching you with His divine presence. It is remembrance that increases faith.

Chapter excerpted from Julia Loren, *Divine Intervention: True Stories of Heaven Invading Earth* (Reading, CA: Tharseo Publishing, 2008), foreword.

About the Author

Bill Johnson is the senior pastor of Bethel Church in Redding, California (www.ibethel.org), and the author of several classic books on faith and healing, such as *When Heaven Invades Earth*, *The Supernatural Power of the Transformed Mind*, and *Hosting the Presence*.

THE COMPASSION OF CHRIST
HEALS EVERYONE

F. F. Bosworth

3

THE COMPASSION OF CHRIST HEALS EVERYONE

F. F. Bosworth

Now, since God heals us by sending His Word (see Psalm 107:20), what can be more His Word than His redemptive and covenant names, which were given, all seven of them, for the specific purpose of revealing to every man in Adam's race His redemptive attitude toward them?

When Christ commands us to *"preach the gospel to every creature"* (Mark 16:15), He intends for us to tell the Good News of redemption. His seven redemptive names reveal what our redemption includes. He has many other names, but only seven *redemptive* names, and these seven names are never used in the Scriptures except in His dealings with man. There are not six names, or eight, but seven, the perfect number, because He is a perfect Savior, and His redemption covers the whole scope of human need. The blessings revealed by each of these names are all in the Atonement. For instance,

JEHOVAH-SHAMMAH means *"The LORD is there"* (Ezekiel 48:35), or present, *"made nigh by the blood of Christ"* (Ephesians 2:13).

JEHOVAH-SHALOM is translated "The Lord Our Peace." This is in the Atonement because *"the chastisement of our peace was upon him"* (Isaiah 53:5).

JEHOVAH-RA-AH is translated *"The LORD is my shepherd"* (Psalm 23:1). He became our Shepherd by giving His life for the sheep. (See John 10:11, 15.) So, you see, this privilege is in the Atonement.

JEHOVAH-JIREH means "The Lord Will Provide" an offering (see Genesis 22:8)—Christ Himself being the Offering provided on Calvary.

He became JEHOVAH-NISSI, "The Lord our Banner," or "Victor," by *"spoil[ing] principalities and powers"* on the cross (Colossians 2:15).

He bore our sins and became JEHOVAH-TSIDKENU, *"THE LORD OUR RIGHTEOUSNESS"* (Jeremiah 23:6), opening the way for every sinner to receive the gift of righteousness.

JEHOVAH-RAPHA is translated *"I am the LORD that healeth thee"* (Exodus 15:26), or "I am the Lord your Physician." This also is in the Atonement, for *"Himself took our infirmities, and bare our sicknesses"* (Matthew 8:17).

This completes the list of the seven redemptive names, which were given for the purpose of revealing God's relationship toward us all under each of these seven titles. These seven names all belong abidingly to Christ, and it is under each of these seven titles that He is the same yesterday, today and forever. (See Hebrews 13:8.) Jesus says to all who come to Him for any of these seven blessings, *"Him that cometh to me I will in no wise cast out"* (John 6:37).

This is the Good News that God wants preached to every creature, so that every creature may have the privilege of enjoying *"the fulness of the blessing of the gospel of Christ"* (Romans 15:29).

I say again that nothing is more God's Word *"settled in heaven"* (Psalm 119:89) than His redemptive name JEHOVAH-RAPHA. No one has a right to change God's "I *am* JEHOVAH-RAPHA" to "I *was* JEHOVAH-RAPHA" because *"the word of the Lord endureth for ever"* (1 Peter 1:25).

Since JEHOVAH-SHALOM, "The Lord Our Peace," is one of Christ's redemptive names, has not every man a redemptive right to obtain peace from Him? Has not every man, likewise, a redemptive right to obtain victory from Jehovah-nissi? Has not every man a redemptive right to obtain *"the gift of righteousness"* (Romans 5:17) from Jehovah-tsidkenu, and so forth? If so, why has not every man a redemptive right to obtain healing from Jehovah-rapha?

This name, Jehovah-rapha, was so accepted and believed by those to whom it was first sent that *"there was not one feeble person among their tribes"* (Psalm 105:37); and whenever this state of health was interfered with by their transgressions, as soon as they repented, typical atonements were made, and God was still Jehovah-rapha, the Healer, not to some, but to all. God wants this redemptive name, as well as all the others, to be sent *"to every creature"* (Mark 16:15), with the promise that *"they shall recover"* (Mark 16:18), for *"the Lord shall raise [them] up"* (James 5:15).

⁓

Jesus Healed Everything and Everyone

*And Jesus went about all Galilee, teaching...and preaching the gospel... and healing **all manner** of sickness and **all manner** of disease among the people. And his fame went throughout all Syria: and they brought unto him all sick people that were taken with divers diseases and torments, and those which were possessed with devils, and those which were lunatic, and those that had the palsy; and he healed them ["all" moffatt]. And there followed him great multitudes of people from Galilee, and from Decapolis, and from Jerusalem, and from Judaea, and from beyond Jordan.* (Matthew 4:23–25)

And Jesus went about all the cities and villages, teaching...and preaching the gospel...and healing every sickness and every disease among the people. But when he saw the multitudes, he was moved with compassion on them....And when he had called unto him his twelve disciples, he gave them power against unclean spirits, to cast them out, and to heal all manner of sickness and all manner of disease. (Matthew 9:35–36; 10:1)

Note that it was the multitudes coming for healing that necessitated the thrusting forth of new laborers into His harvest to preach and to heal. It was not long until seventy more were needed, and were sent forth to heal as well as to preach. Let us look at several more Scriptures that show that Jesus healed everyone who came to Him for healing:

Jesus…withdrew himself from thence: and great multitudes followed him, and he healed them all.   (Matthew 12:15)

And Jesus went forth, and saw a great multitude, and was moved with compassion toward them, and he healed their sick.   (Matthew 14:14)

And when [Jesus and His disciples] were gone over, they came into the land of Gennesaret. And when the men of that place had knowledge of him, they sent out into all that country round about, and brought unto him all that were diseased; and besought him that they might only touch the hem of his garment: and as many as touched were made perfectly whole.   (Matthew 14:34–36)

A great multitude of people out of all Judaea and Jerusalem, and from the sea coast of Tyre and Sidon, which came to hear him, and to be healed of their diseases; and they that were vexed with unclean spirits: and they were healed. And the whole multitude sought to touch him: for there went virtue out of him, and healed them all.   (Luke 6:17–19)

We see throughout the Gospels that, in bringing the sick to Christ for healing, it was repeatedly stated that *all* the sick were brought, which included all the "unlucky" ones whom it was supposedly not God's will to heal, if there were any. If, according to modern tradition, it is God's will for the sick to patiently remain so for His glory, is it not strange that there should not be even one of this type of person in all these multitudes who were brought to Christ for healing? By healing the epileptic (see Mark 9:14–29), Jesus proved it to be the Father's will to heal even this one whom the disciples, divinely commissioned to cast out demons, failed to deliver. We see by this passage that it would have been wrong to call into question God's willingness to heal, and to teach it, because of this failure on the part of the disciples. Jesus, by healing him, showed them that the failure to heal proved nothing but unbelief. Peter, after three years of constant association with the Lord, described His earthly ministry in this one brief statement: *"God anointed Jesus of Nazareth with the Holy Ghost and with power: who went about doing good, and healing all that were oppressed of the devil; for God was with him"* (Acts 10:38).

So, in all the above Scriptures, and in many others that show He healed all the sick, we have the will of God revealed for our bodies, and the answer to the question, Is healing for all?

⌒

Christ's Continuing Ministry of Healing

Many in our day have been taught that Christ performed miracles of healing just to show His power and to prove His deity. This may be true, but it is far from being all the truth. He would not have had to heal *all* to show His power; a few outstanding cases would have proven this. But the Scriptures show that He healed because of His compassion and to fulfill prophecy. Others teach that He healed the sick to make Himself known, but in Matthew 12:15–16, we read, *"Great multitudes followed him, and he healed them all; and charged them that they should **not make him known**."*

Some who have to admit that Jesus healed all who came to Him hold that Isaiah's prophecy concerning His bearing of our sicknesses refers only to His earthly ministry, that this universal manifestation of His compassion was special and not a revelation of the unchanging will of God. But the Bible clearly teaches that He only *"began both to do and teach"* (Acts 1:1) what was not only to be continued, but augmented, after His ascension.

After Christ, for three years, had healed all who came to Him, He said, *"It is expedient* [profitable] *for you that I go away"* (John 16:7). How could this be true if His going away would modify His ministry to the afflicted?

Anticipating the unbelief with which this wonderful promise would be regarded, He prefaced His promise to continue the same and *"greater works"* in answer to our prayers after His exaltation, with the words *"verily, verily"*:

*Verily, verily, I say unto you, he that believeth on me, the works that I do shall he do also; and greater works than these shall he do; because I go unto my Father. And [how are we to do them?] whatsoever ye shall ask in my name, that will **I** do, that the Father may be glorified in the Son.*
(John 14:12–13)

In other words, we are to do them by asking *Him* to do them.

He did not say "less works," but *"the works"* and *"greater works."*

To me, this promise from the lips of Christ is a complete answer to all opposers and to all their books and articles against divine healing.

"It is written" was Christ's policy when resisting the Devil. (See, for example, Matthew 4:4.)

William Jennings Bryan well asked, "Since Christ said 'It is written,' and the devil said 'It is written,' why can't the preacher say 'It is written'?"

The Wisdom of the Early Church

The early church took Christ at His word and prayed unitedly for signs and wonders of healing, until *"the place was shaken where they were assembled together"* (Acts 4:31); and then

they brought forth the sick into the streets, and laid them on beds and couches....There came also a multitude out of the cities round about unto Jerusalem, bringing sick folks, and them which were vexed with unclean spirits: and they were healed every one. (Acts 5:15–16)

The Gospels describe *"all that Jesus **began** both to do and teach"* (Acts 1:1). In this incident in the book of Acts, Jesus was continuing His ministry from the right hand of God through His *"body, the church"* (Colossians 1:18), according to His promise. Some say, "Oh, that was only in the beginning of the Acts of the Apostles, for the purpose of confirming their word regarding Christ's resurrection."

Let us, then, turn to the *last* chapter of Acts, and read how, thirty years later, after Paul, on the island of Melita, had healed the father of

Publius, *"all the other sick people in the island came and were cured"* (Acts 28:9 WEY).

So we see again, even at this time, in the very last chapter of the Acts of the Holy Spirit, which is the only unfinished book of the New Testament, it was still the will of God to heal not some, but all.

Journey into Word & Spirit

1. What are your thoughts about Jesus' desire and ability to heal you?

2. What hinders you from daring to believe that Jesus is full of compassion and love toward you even now?

3. Have you ever seen or heard of someone being healed by the power of Jesus? Describe what happened.

Chapter compiled from F. F. Bosworth, *Christ the Healer* (New Kensington, PA: Whitaker House, 2000), 53–56, 59–61, 102–104.

About the Author

F. F. Bosworth (1877–1958) strongly influenced many of the early healing evangelists, including Oral Roberts, T. L. Osborn, John G. Lake, and many others. He worked with renowned healer John Alexander Dowie for a number of years before starting his own healing ministry. First published in 1924, Bosworth's book *Christ the Healer* is a tremendous work on the principles of healing through the finished work of Christ on the cross at Calvary.

GRABBING HOLD OF GOD

Mark Stibbe

4

GRABBING HOLD OF GOD

Mark Stibbe

*"Laying hold upon God is not the act of a dead man,
neither is it the deed of one who is destitute of spiritual perception;
it is the act of one who is quickened and kept alive
by the indwelling power of the Holy Spirit."*
—Charles Spurgeon

I noticed it because I love soccer and I am always on the lookout for testimonies of healing.

It was all over our very secular British newspapers at the end of the 2005 season. The story concerned a soccer player called Marvin Andrews who played for Glasgow Rangers, one of the most successful Scottish teams in recent decades. The reports in the newspapers ran the headline, "The Miracle of Marvin Andrews' Knee." That caught my attention.

Marvin Andrews scored the winning goal on the last day of the season to secure not just victory on the day but the title for the whole season. At the end of the match he knelt down in the centre circle of the pitch to pray and give thanks to the Lord. On his T-shirt the crowd could read words from Luke's Gospel, "The things that are impossible with [men] are possible with God."

Why did Marvin make such a gesture? In a match against Dundee a month before, Andrews had ruptured his anterior cruciate ligament—a 35mm link at the knee between the femur and tibia that provides stability and balance. This is an injury that can end a player's career. The Rangers medical staff told Marvin that he would need surgery followed by months of rehabilitation. But he refused to have the operation and chose instead to go to God in prayer. "I prayed to God," he said, "and he spoke. God is not deaf. He speaks. Some people cannot believe it; they think he doesn't reply. But my God is not like that. When I speak to him he replies. God told me not to have the operation."

Needless to say, those advising Marvin were appalled. The medical staff told him that he had to have the operation or his career would be over. Marvin comments, "Doubts came, fear came, the devil tried to bring fear into me, just as the Bible said. There were all different kinds of people speaking negatively, speaking fear into me, but I kept holding on to God. This is what faith is about. God kept telling me, 'Keep believing, keep trusting.' And that gave me strength."

Against all odds, within three weeks Marvin Andrews was back playing football. He played the last four games of the season and helped Rangers win the title. His manager Alex McLeish stated, "Marvin is defying logic." Marvin himself said this—and this was reported in the national newspapers of Great Britain:

I'm a servant of the Lord. I'm here to tell people that he is still alive, that we still have the same God that opened the blind eyes and allowed the crippled man to walk. I'm here to continue proclaiming the gospel, to tell people the good news.

The Importance of Faith

[There are many] Gospel episodes where Jesus takes the initiative and touches the lives of the sick, bringing miraculous healing....We looked at examples of this royal initiative today—ways in which God has stretched out his hand and healed sick people in the most extraordinary ways. Sometimes this happens immediately—without human intermediary; sometimes it happens in a mediated way, with a believer administering the touch that changes everything.

All this emphasis on God's sovereign touch is good news. At the same time it can become bad news if we're not careful. It can give us cause to become passive. In other words, people who over-emphasise the doctrine of the sovereignty of God can very easily slip into a resignation which looks like determinism. "Well, God is sovereign. If he is going to heal me, he'll do it without any help from me." This almost feels like a "Que sera, sera" mentality—"Whatever will be, will be."

Now of course we have to be wise here. God is indeed sovereign and... he is perfectly capable of making his move independently of us. All this has ample biblical precedent in those stories where Jesus touches those who are not actively involved in their healing. The best example is...the raising of the widow's boy at Nain. The boy was dead and of course played no part at all in his miracle. He was 100 percent passive in the process.

At the same time we mustn't stop there. There are not just stories in the Gospels where Jesus touches those in need. There are also episodes where sick people play an active and almost aggressive part in touching Jesus. In these incidents, people who are absolutely desperate pursue the person of Jesus with a deep and unbridled sense of abandonment. In these situations it seems almost as if it is their faith that secures the healing. In these instances, grabbing hold of Jesus seems to be the critical factor in determining the outcome they desired. They run hard after the King in order to reach out and touch him, and as they do so, it changes everything in their world.

All this highlights the human part played in miracles. Miracles are always the result of God's will, yes. But they also occur in environments where someone has real faith. The reason why I like Marvin Andrews' testimony is because it is the testimony of a man who believed that nothing is impossible for God, who grabbed hold of God's promises and continued to exercise faith even when others were speaking negatively to him. That is not passivity! That is not a deterministic "Whatever will be, will be." That is faith.

The Woman Who Touched the King

You may have anticipated the incident I am going to describe now. Mark talks about it in chapter 5 of his Gospel, Matthew in chapter 9 and Luke in chapter 8. Jesus is on his way to the house of a synagogue ruler called Jairus, whose 12-year-old daughter is very sick. The dad manages to get Jesus to come to his house. On the way Jesus is delayed by the conduct of a woman desperate for healing. Luke records the incident as follows:

> *Now a woman, having a flow of blood for twelve years, who had spent all her livelihood on physicians and could not be healed by any, came from behind and touched the border of His garment. And immediately her flow of blood stopped. And Jesus said, "Who touched Me?" When all denied it, Peter and those with him said, "Master, the multitudes throng and press You, and You say, 'Who touched Me?'" But Jesus said, "Somebody touched Me, for I perceived power going out from Me." Now when the woman saw that she was not hidden, she came trembling; and falling down before Him, she declared to Him in the presence of all the people the reason she had touched Him and how she was healed immediately. And He said to her, "Daughter, be of good cheer; your faith has made you well. Go in peace."* (Luke 8:43–48 NKJV)

There are many things that are important to notice about this incident. I'd like to point to five in particular.

First, note the way in which Luke emphasises the power of just one touch in this episode. Five times he uses the verb *haptomai*, to touch, in the report of this incident. Luke was a physician. As a medic he seems fascinated by the healing effects of touching the King. All the woman did was touch Jesus, and this changed absolutely everything. This fact alone clearly intrigues Dr. Luke.

The second thing we should note is that the woman was "unclean." Her bleeding disorder made her impure in the eyes of the Rabbis. Yet Jesus does not condemn her for touching him, nor does he believe himself unclean. Jesus touches the "untouchables," and the "untouchables" touch Jesus. Indeed, he goes on to Jairus' house to touch the girl who is now dead.

That brings me thirdly to the mention of "twelve years." (See Luke 8:42.) The girl was twelve years old. The woman had had the bleeding disorder for twelve years. This means that the girl was born in the year that the woman began to suffer from her infirmity. This sounds like another example of "Kingdom synchronicity." These two lives—joined by the number of years mentioned—are wonderfully transformed on the very same day.

The fourth thing to note is the way that Jesus stops a whole crowd for just one person. There was a sense of urgency, at least in Jairus. He wanted to get Jesus to his daughter as soon as he possibly could. But when the woman touched Jesus, he stopped the entire procession in order to find out who it was. That speaks to me of the profound compassion of Jesus. He did not live by the tyranny of the urgent. He lived a life of love.

The final thing I want to mention is the woman's faith. She had spent all her money on consulting medics, and they had not managed to cure her problem. It would have been possible for her at this point to say, "I am going to have to live with this. It must be God's will." But she does not. Hearing that Jesus is in town, she pursues him through the crowd, desperate to touch the garment of the King. Why does she do that? What is going on in her heart? The only thing we can say is that she must have heard the testimonies of Jesus' healing miracles and that faith—which comes by hearing—has welled up in her heart.

Faith means "believing what you cannot see." Or, as St. Augustine said, "Faith is to believe what we do not see; the reward of faith is to see what we believe." The woman cannot see her healing. Yet she believes that she is going to receive it. So she presses in and grabs hold of the Royal Healer and in doing so she is *immediately* healed. Jesus' words conclude the story: *"Your faith has made you well."* Matthew Henry puts it very compassionately:

> Her faith was very strong; for she doubted not but that by the touch of the hem of his garment she should derive from him healing virtue sufficient for her relief, looking upon him to be such a full fountain of mercies that she should steal a cure and he not miss it. Thus many a poor soul is healed, and helped, and saved, by Christ, that is lost in a crowd, and that nobody takes notice of.

However hard we try, we cannot escape the importance of faith in this passage. Like Marvin Andrews, the woman in Luke 8 has heard many unpromising things from the medics in her life and yet she chooses to believe that Jesus has the power to heal her. That implies at least some human part in the healing event. Some of course will argue that faith is a divine gift and that her belief in Jesus' power was inspired by God. Even if that's true in this case, the woman still had to co-operate with God. She was not a robot programmed to believe. She was not compelled to run hard after the Healer. She chose to be active in the process. She made the decision to put her trust in Jesus and to believe that nothing is too hard for the Lord. In a time of extreme trouble, she pushed past all her doubts and fears and broke into the presence of her Deliverer. No wonder Jesus applauded her faith.

The Hem of Jesus' Garment

But what was her faith in, exactly? To answer that question we need to understand the Jewish background to the story. In particular, we need to understand why it is that the woman touches "the hem of Jesus' garment." What did Luke mean by this phrase?

In Jesus' day, Jewish men wore a woollen outer garment called the *tallit*. On each of the four corners of this garment there were tassels known as *tzitzit*. These *tzitzit* were extremely important for religious reasons. They were worn in accordance with Numbers 15:37–40, where the Lord tells Moses to instruct his people to make tassels to wear on their garments for all future generations. These tassels were to be a reminder of all the commandments of the Lord, a stimulus to obey all that God required to live a holy life.

According to Jewish expert Dwight Pryor, the *tzitzit* had a specific design. Each tassel consisted of eight strands of thread. Four strands (three white and one blue) were looped through an opening in the corner of the garment and then folded over to become eight in total. These eight strands were then tied in a series of five double knots.

All of this was extremely important in terms of symbolism. The five knots were a reminder of the Torah, which consisted of the first five books of the Bible. The four strands were a reminder of the Tetragrammaton, the four Greek letters that made up the sacred covenant name for God revealed to Moses (YHWH). The number 13 (8+5) was a reminder of the oneness of God. The word *echad* in Hebrew has the numeric value of 13, and this word means "one," as in "the Lord is one" (i.e., indivisible). The word *tzitzit* itself has a numerical value of 600, which, when added to the 13 already stated above, makes 613. In Jewish tradition there were 613 commandments in the five books of the Torah.

The tassels on Jesus' outer garment were therefore extremely rich in terms of their symbolism. They stood for the sacred name of God (the four strands), the instructions of God (the five double knots), the oneness of God (the eight strands tied in five double knots) and the totality of God's commandments (600+13).

According to a Jewish interpretation of this passage, the woman was expressing faith in God in the fullest sense. She was not directing her faith towards some supposed mystical properties in the tassels themselves. That would have been superstition. Rather, she was reaching out to the wholeness of who God is, and in the process she experienced wholeness! As Dwight Pryor puts it, she was effectively saying, "If I can but lay hold of the totality or the fullness of God: who he is; his nature, his word and his will—i.e., if I can but touch the wholeness of God—I myself can be made whole" (www.jcstudies.com). Now that's what I call "faith."

The Kingdom Is for the Desperate

One of my great heroes is George Muller, who built orphanages in Bristol during the nineteenth century. He lived entirely by faith and said this: "Faith does not operate in the realm of the possible. There is no glory for God in that which is humanly possible. Faith begins where man's power ends."

This kind of faith is often vital for receiving the touch of the King that changes everything. A holy desperation is required if we are to persevere and see the breakthroughs we long for. Passive faith (which is really a contradiction in terms) will not do. Scepticism is not helpful. What is needed is active, living, dynamic faith that springs from a passionate pursuit of God.

The great revival theologian Jonathan Edwards had a great name for this kind of thing. He called it "pressing into the Kingdom of God." In a sermon with that same title Edwards once defined what he meant:

Pressing into the kingdom of heaven denotes earnestness and firmness of resolution. There should be strength of resolution, accompanying strength of desire, as it was in the psalmist: "one thing have I desired, and that will I seek after."

Edwards went on to say:

There are two things needful in a person, in order to possess these strong resolutions; there must be a sense of the great importance and necessity of the mercy sought, and there must also be a sense of opportunity to obtain it, or the encouragement there is to seek it.

While Edwards did not believe that divine healing was available in his own day, his principles are still relevant. The woman in Luke 8 was certainly earnest and firm in her resolution. Furthermore, the woman had both necessity and opportunity. She desperately needed healing and she saw in Jesus the opportunity of her healing. The Kingdom of God is truly for the desperate.

Helen's Story

About ten years ago I invited Bishop Joseph and Pastor Barbara Garlington over to the church I was then leading, St. Andrew's Chorleywood. They minister in Pittsburgh in a wonderful growing and vibrant church. They brought their choir over with them, and we had an extraordinary weekend in the presence of God together, worshipping, listening to great teaching and going to the next level in our walk with God.

One of the many people in our church transformed by this visit was a young woman called Helen, a theology graduate who had experienced major illness and disability in her time at university. Desperate for healing, she pressed through the crowds in our church on the Sunday morning to ask Pastor Barbara (who heads up the healing ministry at their church in Pittsburgh) to pray for her. Helen tells the story in her own words:

When I was 21, in my final year of university, I had to have spine surgery, and during my recovery I found out that I was partially deaf in both ears. This knocked me for six as I had just had eight months of real hardship, and then to find this out really tested my faith and dependency on God.

I was very tired of dealing with things so just accepted it. When Mark Stibbe gave a talk on being desperate for God's healing touch, I had no idea how to be desperate. The exhaustion and emotional numbness far exceeded my ability to seek healing actively. It was as if I was resigned to the fact that I had this disability. I had to wear a hearing aid for eighteen months—which I hated; it was only in one ear, so my hearing still wasn't good and it was very frustrating for me and everyone around me.

Then my tinnitus (which I have had for as long as I can remember) got worse and was constant rather than being intermittent. It was stopping me from sleeping, from concentrating at work, from relaxing; it gave me headaches and I was getting exhausted and full of resentment.

Then came the church weekend when Bishop Joseph and Pastor Barbara Garlington came to our church at St. Andrew's. I went to the Friday evening service when the choir from Pittsburgh were singing and just broke down. The exhaustion, the frustration, the headaches had all got too much for me and I just cried. This for me is rather unusual, as I am not a particularly emotional person—especially in public—but I just didn't care, I had had too much.

On the Saturday night I said to God, "If you want me to go to church on Sunday morning then you had better wake me up." At 10:30 a.m. I woke up and decided that it was not enough time to get ready and stayed in bed. My mum came home from the 9:00 service and challenged me about going, so I went, and Bishop Joseph was talking about being expectant for God's favour. I got really into this and was waiting for the prayer ministry at the end, but there wasn't any. I just couldn't believe it. I am no good at going up for prayer, and the one day that I actually wanted to, there wasn't any.

However, I saw Pastor Barbara and I wanted her to pray for me, so I fought the typically British attitude of reserve and found myself walking over to her, not tentatively, but as though nothing was going to prevent me from knocking on God's door about this. I was that desperate. I asked her if she was in a hurry, and she said no, so I outlined why I was here and how cross I was that there was no ministry. So she prayed for me, and for the first time in a long time, the Holy Spirit moved visibly and powerfully on my life. With me he is normally gentle, but not this time. We were waging war together. My attitude towards it was, "Well, God, I have nothing left, I cannot cope any more; you have to move now." I am never this assertive but it just didn't seem like there was any option other than God healing me. And he did!

When I relayed this story to my mother she was astounded at me, not because God had healed me, but because I had stepped that far out of character. My desperation led me to obedience and the expectation that God would move. But the flipside of it was that I was fully ready to accept the healing—no doubts, no nonsense—and I think that is why my hearing got better and better the more people I told. The more people I told, the clearer my hearing got, and now I don't use my hearing aid and have very little problem hearing people. I praise God for what he has done.

What Is Faith?

Helen showed great faith in that story. But what, then, is faith? This is a question asked by the writer of the Letter to the Hebrews. He begins chapter 11 with these words, "What is faith? It is the confident assurance that what we hope for is going to happen. It is the evidence of things we cannot yet see" (NLT). How do we come to have such faith?

There are two views here. The first says that this kind of faith is a gift. The thinking behind this is that there are three types of faith talked about in the New Testament. There is first of all what I call "conversion" faith. This is the faith I had back in 1977 when I confessed my sins and declared that I believed that Jesus is my Saviour, Lord, and Friend. On that day way back in 1977 I was justified by faith. I was made right with God by believing in what

Jesus Christ has accomplished at the Cross. That is what I mean by "conversion" faith. You can't become a Christian without it.

But then there is a second kind of faith talked about in the New Testament. I call this "continuing" faith. When I became a Christian I chose to believe in Jesus. But that was not the end of the matter as regards faith. I have to go on believing in Jesus every day. I need continuing faith, not just conversion faith.

Then thirdly there is what I call "charismatic" faith. If you remember the list of the spiritual gifts in 1 Corinthians 12..., you will notice that Paul mentions faith as a charismatic or grace gift in verses 8–11. He qualifies what this kind of faith is at the start of 1 Corinthians 13 when he describes a faith "that can move mountains." Charismatic faith is mountain-moving faith. It is a sudden, supernatural surge of confidence that God is going to do something miraculous. It might be the conversion of someone whom we thought would never come to Christ. It might be the healing of someone whom we thought was beyond help. It might be the rescue of a marriage that we considered irreparable. God gives "charismatic" faith to certain individuals in his church when he is about to move a mountain of impossibility.

A few moments ago I asked the question, "How do we come to have the kind of faith that constitutes 'confident assurance that what we hope for is going to happen'?" The first answer to this question is that we need to pray for the spiritual gift of faith. When it comes to the miraculous and life-changing touch of the King, charismatic (rather than merely continuing) faith is required, and this is a gift to be received, not a feeling you can just whip up.

The second answer to the question is that this kind of special faith is something we exercise according to our own choice and initiative. In this way of thinking, faith is something we decide and discipline ourselves to develop over time. It is "continuing" faith exercised at a higher level. The passage often used to support this view is Mark 4:26–29 (NKJV):

And He said, "The kingdom of God is as if a man should scatter seed on the ground, and should sleep by night and rise by day, and the seed should sprout and grow, he himself does not know how. For the earth yields crops by itself: first the blade, then the head, after that the full grain in the head.

But when the grain ripens, immediately he puts in the sickle, because the harvest has come."

Those who believe that special or dynamic faith is something we can all exercise point to the growth of the seed here: first the blade, then the head, then the full grain in the head. They liken faith to the seed. It is supposed to develop, strengthen, and grow. To put it another way, faith is like a muscle. It is something we exercise, and the more we exercise it, the stronger it becomes.

So there are two views that I routinely come across when it comes to faith (understood as the confident assurance that a thing hoped for is going to occur). The first says that this kind of faith is a gift supernaturally and suddenly bestowed by God. The second says that it is something we choose to exercise in a given situation of need and challenge.

A Fighting Faith

The argument over which of these two views is correct will no doubt continue. In the end, however, one thing is certain, that it is impossible to please God without faith (Hebrews 11:6). All Christians are called to exercise faith. All Christians are called on a daily basis to believe in what they cannot yet see—to put their trust in invisible Kingdom realities. More than that, the majority of great breakthroughs in the Christian life occur when someone somewhere has exercised what I call "fighting faith." Like Helen in the testimony, they have pursued God with desperation. They have been aggressive, active, and determined in their exercise of faith. Helen's story shows that breakthroughs come when a fighting faith has been displayed. As Ralph Erskine says, "Faith, without trouble or fighting, is a suspicious faith; for true faith is a fighting, wrestling faith."

In County Armagh in Northern Ireland, a woman called Sharyn Mackay was diagnosed with cancer and told that she had twelve months to live. This mother of four was informed that she had a rare form of cancer that had spread to her lungs and her kidneys. She was told that it was certain she was going to die. Sharyn was devastated by the news. Only the day before, she had celebrated the birthday of one of her children. Now she was being told that she wouldn't live to see the next one.

Sharyn knew that only her Christian faith could help her now. This was all that was left. At this point she heard about some healing meetings that were going on in the Solihull Renewal Centre in England. These meetings were being hosted by Dr. David Carr.... Sharyn and her husband William decided they would go. This is how she describes what happened:

As soon as we entered the building we felt an enormous heat. It was as though there was an incredible presence in the room and an overwhelming feeling of love. As soon as the meeting finished I felt as though the cancer had left my body.

On Friday 8 July 2004 Sharyn and William set off for their hospital to get the latest results. They prayed all the way there, and though naturally very anxious they felt a supernatural peace. When the consultant came in he was smiling. He said, "Sharyn, you are going to leave the hospital happier than when you came in." He told Sharyn that she wasn't going to die, because every trace of cancer had completely disappeared. Four radiographers had pored over her test results and were astonished to find no cancer in Sharyn's lungs or kidneys. They had no explanation for it.

The couple were overjoyed at this news. Since then they have started their own healing ministry and now encourage other people to believe in the power of prayer. More than that, Sharyn's miraculous recovery has become well known in Northern Ireland, where it is now being taught as part of the curriculum in schools as an example of a modern-day miracle!

What an example of "fighting faith." Fighting faith is not faith without anxiety or tears. Fighting faith is a faith that pushes through walls of doubt and fear to a place of breakthrough. Fighting faith is what Sharyn exhibited. Fighting faith is what we see in Helen's story. If you ask me whether this kind of faith is divine or human, I would have to say it's both! It's a gift from God, something donated by our loving Heavenly Father. But it is also something that we have to act upon courageously and intentionally. Faith—particularly fighting faith—is a vital ingredient in the King's touch. Fighting faith seizes hold of Jesus when opportunity knocks.

When the King Passes By

Someone once said that the opportunity of a lifetime must be seized in the lifetime of the opportunity. There are moments in the Gospels when the King of kings is passing by and people seize the moment. Not only do they seize the moment, they grab hold of the King. It is as if something deep within their hearts knows that just one touch from this King will change everything.

I wonder whether you have ever been in a situation where you had a once-in-a-lifetime opportunity to shake the hand of someone really famous, someone really influential, someone you respected for their position in life. That happened to a friend J.John and me. We were in Washington, D.C., and had the opportunity of going not just to the White House on a tour but into the West Wing for lunch with several Christians who worked for President George W. Bush. We had a great time. Deep down, however, we were both very keen to bump into the President. We wanted to shake hands with him, not because we are closet Republicans but because we knew he was a man of faith and because we knew it would give us a great story!

Well, we didn't see the President during the tour of the West Wing or during lunch in the West Wing Mess. After our meal we left the table, and both of us went to the rest room. Once inside we realised we were the only people there. We had seen all the secret agents dressed in black suits and talking into concealed microphones, so we decided to have some fun. We pretended to be secret agents ourselves, talking into our sleeves as we washed and dried our hands. We had a great laugh at the expense of these gentlemen, not realising that they were probably watching us on hidden cameras and having a laugh at our expense too!

As a result of all this childish humour we were longer than we should have been. When we came out, the two men who had been escorting us round the West Wing looked at us in despair. They knew how keen we had been to shake hands with the President. Well, while we were wasting time pretending to be secret servicemen, the President and the Vice-President had walked past on the way to the situation room. They had stopped to shake the hands of the two gentlemen looking after us. If we had not been play-acting, we too would have been there and would have been able to shake hands with the most powerful man on the planet!

Ever since that moment I have used that story—at my own expense—to encourage people not to waste their opportunity to reach out for the hand of the King. The trouble is there are too many Christians messing around in the rest room when the King of kings is passing by.

A *Diasozo* Move of God

In the Gospels, we see individuals grabbing hold of their opportunity when Jesus passes by. Desperate for just one touch, they reach out to him and find their healing. They don't mess around. They don't waste time. They seize the opportunity of a lifetime in the lifetime of that opportunity.

This happens in the case of individuals, such as the woman with the bleeding disorder. This also happens with whole crowds of people. In fact, one of my favourite examples of this is right at the end of Matthew 14. The disciples have just crossed the lake and arrive at Gennesaret with Jesus. Matthew records that:

> *When they had crossed over, they came to the land of Gennesaret. And when the men of that place recognized Him, they sent out into all that surrounding region, brought to Him all who were sick, and begged Him that they might only touch the hem of His garment. And as many as touched it were made perfectly well.* (Matthew 14:34–36 NKJV)

Twice Matthew uses the verb *haptomai*, to touch, in this report. Here we have not just individuals touching Jesus. We have a large number of people touching him.

What characterised all of these people in their desire to touch Jesus? The answer is simple: it was fighting faith. These people really believed that Jesus could change their situation. They believed that if they could get close enough to him, if they could just touch him, then blind eyes would see, deaf ears would hear, lame legs would be healed, tumours would fall off, and so on. They all had one thing besides sickness in common: they had FAITH. They really believed in Jesus' power to save, heal, and deliver.

And so Matthew reports that they were healed. The word in the original Greek is actually a lot more exciting. Instead of the usual Greek verb for heal, *sozo*, Matthew uses a much rarer word, *diasozo*. This is a combination of *sozo*, to heal, and *dia*, meaning thoroughly or completely. *Diasozo* means to cure completely, to restore perfectly, to heal totally. What Matthew is talking about here is total cures. In Gennesaret, the crowds reached out to Jesus and just one touch changed everything—totally, perfectly, completely.

Don't you just long for a *diasozo* move of God like that today? For that to happen, we will need to be desperate enough to grab hold of the King as he passes by. In short, we will need to have faith in God. We will need to have fighting faith.

Time to Reach Out to Jesus

In 2005 I was preaching on the subject…: "One touch from the King changes everything." As we started to sing a song of worship, a lady on the front row was reflecting on this idea of the King's transforming touch. She had a serious disability caused by a horrific car accident twenty years earlier. As a result of her injuries she had not been able to lift her left hand above the level of her shoulder for two decades. Her left arm was locked in position, as if it was in a sling.

Remembering the story of the woman reaching out to touch Jesus' garment, she decided that she was going to reach out to God. Desperate for her healing, she started to sing praises to the Lord and stretch out her disabled arm to heaven. Suddenly she found she was able to do what she'd been unable to do since her accident. She raised her left hand so that her arm was completely outstretched above her head. For the first time in two decades she was able to raise both arms in adoration. As she did so, her husband standing next to her saw what was happening and fell to his seat, weeping.

No one had asked her to come to the front to receive. No one was praying for her at the time with the laying-on of hands. She simply reached out to touch the King. Two days later she shared her testimony with the whole church. The church family—who knew the lady well—broke into applause and shared in her joy.

I love the way Bishop Joseph Garlington puts it in his amazing song "Just One Touch":

> This is your moment; don't wait
> This is your hour; press in
> Only reach out; it's time to receive
> Look to me now and only believe.

I believe God is calling those in need to stretch out their hand to touch the King and to do so with fighting faith. I also believe that God is calling those who pray for the sick to do so with the same kind of fighting faith.

Only this morning I received an email from two of our missionaries working in Eastern Europe. They reported the following incident:

> *We went out on Sunday to a town nearby. Our colleagues Mike and Kathryn went too. They decided to leave their two children, James (4) and Elizabeth (3), at home with their babysitter. We had a good day but when we arrived back we got a call from Mike saying that James had fallen and broken his arm at the elbow.*
>
> *It's always a concern when there is any major medical problem here as they are not equipped with facilities or specialist staff. We needed a bone specialist and were not sure if they had one in town. All our missionary doctors were out of town, which is unusual. So Mike took James to a local hospital where they X-rayed his arm and said it was broken. They then put a plaster cast on halfway round the diameter of his arm and sent him home. Mike was told to bring him back the next day and they X-rayed it again, took off the plaster and then put the same plaster back on again. We were not sure what to think of this, but we had to trust God. So the four of us laid hands on James and prayed that God would heal him.*
>
> *This morning, James told his parents that God spoke to him during the night and told him to stretch out his arm and that it was better. Not the normal kind of thing that a four-year-old says. Sure enough, when he got up this morning he was able to use his arm just as normal.*

What God told that four-year-old boy he is telling many others too: "Stretch out your arm."

In Mark chapter 3, Jesus heals a man with a withered arm. Mark reports in verse 5 (NLT): "He said to the man, 'Reach out your hand.' The man reached out his hand, and it became normal again!" The man had to play his part by stretching out his arm in faith and obedience. Jesus then played his part by healing the man miraculously. Healing miracles are God's work, to be sure. But we have a part to play in the process. We are to exhibit fighting faith unless and until we are told otherwise by the Lord.

Journey into Word & Spirit

1. What does "touch the hem of Jesus' garment" mean to you?

2. Is there something God is asking you to do to exhibit "fighting faith"?

Chapter excerpted from Mark Stibbe, *One Touch from the King Changes Everything* (Authentic Media, 2007, 2010), chapter 3, "Grabbing Hold of God." The portion in italics was added by the writer for this publication.

About the Author

Dr. Mark Stibbe is a former British vicar of Saint Andrew's Church, Chorleywood, UK, and is a best-selling author of books on the Father's heart. He founded a media company that helps good writers become great authors, and he is currently writing a series of novels about an eighteenth-century "spy vicar." For more information, please see Mark Stibbe's Web sites, www.thescriptdoctor.org.uk and www.thomaspryce.co.uk, and his author page on www.amazon.com.

HEALING FOR THE BODY

Mary K. Baxter

5

HEALING FOR THE BODY

Mary K. Baxter

*"Beloved, I pray that you may prosper in all things and be in health,
just as your soul prospers."*
—3 John 1:2 (NKJV)

Salvation through Jesus provides us first with healing for our spirits—a new nature, a right relationship with our heavenly Father, and eternal life. Second, it enables us to receive healing for our minds and emotions so that we can be at peace in the midst of life's trials, reflect God's character, and make decisions in line with His Word. Third, it enables us to receive physical healing. *"By His stripes we are healed"* (Isaiah 53:5 NKJV).

An Outpouring of Grace

God has extended many great mercies to me throughout my life. When I reach a point of despair, He always responds with an outpouring of grace. *"From the fullness of his [Jesus'] grace we have all received one blessing after another"* (John 1:16 NIV), and one of those blessings is physical healing.

Once, when I was at home praying, I sensed that something was wrong with one of my children. Sure enough, my son came stumbling through the patio door and collapsed right in front of me! His friends explained that he had been playing football and one of the larger players had accidentally stepped on his head. I immediately called his father at work. He came home, and the two of us rushed our son to the hospital as he was falling into unconsciousness. On the way to the hospital, the car's engine blew up, and by the time we finally got to the hospital, all I could do was cry. I couldn't pray or do anything else.

Some fellow Christians came to the hospital and explained to me that I had lost my faith. Yet, throughout my son's life, he'd been attacked in his head. I was just so tired of the devil attacking my son in this way. On a previous occasion, he'd been ill and we had rushed him to the hospital, where he'd been diagnosed as epileptic.

So, this particular episode, during which his little body had collapsed in front of me, seemed just too much for me. In my desperation, I cried out, *Just take him, God!* After undergoing numerous tests and staying at the hospital all evening, my son regained consciousness. All tests appeared normal, and he was released from the hospital after midnight. Thank the Lord! When we got home, my husband agreed to stay up and watch our son while I went to bed. I went into the bathroom, and the peace of God seemed to overtake me all at once. I got on my knees, and God opened my mouth. Instantly, I thought, *I'm really going to get it from God now because of what I said in that hospital* (telling Him to just take my son). However, it wasn't God's intention to "get me." It was His intention to comfort and heal me.

Weeks earlier, I had gone to the dentist, and as the dentist was working on my teeth, the drill had slipped and flown across the room, so they had left one of my teeth with just a cotton pack in it. I had told my husband, "If God doesn't fill my teeth, then they won't be filled." Well, I had forgotten all about that statement, but God had not forgotten it. He began to fill my teeth in the bathroom after we'd brought my son home from the hospital.

Not once did He rebuke me for telling Him to take my son. Instead, He healed me by filling my teeth! When I finally looked at the clock, I noticed that it was four o'clock in the morning. God had worked on my mouth for four hours. I ran down the hallway and cried out to my husband, "Look, look, God filled my teeth!" He didn't believe it and just told me to go to bed. So, the next morning, I showed him the miracle that God had performed!

As I've ministered the gospel in the United States and overseas, I have encountered this miracle of God many times. He fills people's teeth in order to show them His power. One time, a friend of mine came to my house. She had heard that God was filling teeth in the church services, and she said, "I've got a bad tooth, and I want God to fill it." I said, "Well, I can't guarantee you that God will fill your teeth; it's not me, it's God. I'll pray for you and anoint you, but it has to be God." That night, she actually opened up her mouth like a baby bird, believing that God could fix her tooth. This is faith. She really believed God. The next morning, her tooth was fixed with what looked like white pearl. She told people in various church services that God had fixed her tooth, and when she did, other people's teeth were filled, also. That happens a lot when people get up and testify.

I was preaching at Hudson Bay, Canada, and a lady came up who had about ten cavities. I prayed with her, and she fell on the floor and began to roll, cry, and scream. I thought, *Well, God, I wonder what happened to her?* Later, she got up and came back to me and said, "Look at my mouth." God had filled all her teeth with gold. She explained, "I was shouting with joy and crying because there was no pain at all. I knew what He was doing." I said, "Well, you need to tell people." Yet this woman didn't give her testimony for three years. Then, she came to where I was ministering, and I made her come up and tell the congregation. Many people's teeth were repaired that night because she told what the Lord had done for her.

My mother-in-law had a church in Pennsylvania, and one day, we were praying for people's teeth there. We both saw, in a vision, streams of gold that were about two inches wide. These tiny widths of gold went down and lay in people's teeth where there were cavities, and the angels fixed the people's teeth.

God was showing His power, and it was amazing because one of the people He healed there did not seem to be living for Him and was a hypocrite. But God is merciful.

On another occasion, I was ministering at a church in New York. A woman whose teeth were giving her trouble was the first one to come up to be prayed for that night, and I prayed for her. The next morning, toward the end of the church service, she said, "I have a testimony." I asked her what it was, and she said, "You remember the other night when I couldn't eat because my mouth was hurting too bad? Well, look!" She opened her mouth to reveal the most beautiful fillings. She explained, "I couldn't afford to go to the dentist, and God filled my teeth."

When I was in Malaysia to minister, I met a pastor's wife who asked, "Can you pray for me, because I have a lot of holes in my teeth?" So I placed my hands on her face, and for a while, I could not remove my hands. When I finally finished praying and removed my hands from her face, the holes in her teeth were filled with gold. When God gets ready to show Himself, He does it regardless of what others might think. You have to learn to discern the voice of God because…His ways are not our ways, and His thoughts are not our thoughts.

Another time, I was ministering to about two hundred people in another nation, and I talked about God's miraculous power to fix people's teeth. There was a baby there who was about a year and a half old and was still on milk. The mother had the baby in her arms, and the baby was crying. The child had tiny teeth in front, but some of them were decayed and falling out. The mother said, "The dentist can't do anything." My heart went out to that baby because there's nothing worse than a toothache! I went over and laid hands on the baby, and then I went on down the prayer line. I had prayed for about fifteen other children when the mother screamed. God had healed and regrown all those teeth within fifteen minutes. That was a miracle! Then, many more children's teeth were fixed that day. Little babies don't know what faith is, but children are healed through the love and power of the Lord as we pray for them.

Others have also experienced the healing of their teeth. My friend Pastor Harry Sauer of Faith Fire Word Center in Titusville, Florida, testified,

Mary K. Baxter prayed for my teeth, and I received a gold crown on my left bottom molar. When I went back to the dentist, he asked me what happened because he did not put the crown there. They don't use that quality of gold. I told him I got prayed for and Jesus healed and filled my tooth, praise God!

Another pastor from Independence, Missouri, wrote,

When Sister Baxter came to our church, I had no idea I would receive fillings in my teeth. I had been going to the St. Elizabeth clinic for a few months now for X-rays, cleanings, and extracts. Because they are so busy, my appointments are one to two months apart....But that night, when she called out, "Someone, or there's two of you that have to get fillings, three or four for your teeth," I stood right up; through obedience from the Holy Spirit, I went up to the sanctuary to the sister—and got my silver fillings. I thought I got three, but when I got home, there were three on the left bottom and one on the left top!...What this means to me, though, is that we do definitely serve the same God that raised Lazarus from the dead, the same God that parted the Red Sea when He saved the Israelites,...the God that did a miracle for my daughter and kept her alive....

Twelve Major Miracles

We should never doubt the power of God. On one occasion, my spiritual daughter and I went to a church where the music was so loud that she decided to sit in the back row because her ears were very sensitive. Out of the side door came twelve angels with a long table, and they had twelve transparent boxes with locks on them. I prayed, *Jesus, what's this?* and He replied, *There are going to be twelve major miracles here this morning.* He continued, *Look at the first box.* Locked in the box was a beating heart. The next box held yellow sponges inside it. I thought to myself, *What in the world is that?* The Spirit said, *There are people in here with asthma, and we're going to touch them with these* [items inside the box] *and heal them of their asthma.* There was a kneecap in one box, a nerve in another, and so forth.

I became so overwhelmed that I asked God, *Lord, how am I going to do all this?* So, I called my spiritual daughter from the back of the church to meet me in the corner, and I asked her what she saw. She was a bit hesitant to share it with me at first, but then she went on to describe the same things I'd seen in my vision!

When I stood before the people, the first thing I asked was, "Is there anyone in here who needs healing from asthma or who has bad lungs from smoking?" Immediately, people jumped up and came to the front of the church, and the angels of the Lord took a key, opened that box, and ran over and began touching their lungs. These people fell down on the floor under the power of God and arose healed. One of them even testified, "I saw an angel with a funny object in its hand. I'm embarrassed to tell you what it looked like, but it looked like a sponge." That was yet another confirmation of the vision my daughter and I had seen earlier.

Then, we found out that the pastor of the church needed a heart and that she always walked with a limp from a bad knee. During this service, she, also, fell down under the Spirit of God, and the wings of an angel began to cover her. When she finally got up off the floor, she went to her office weeping. Later, she visited her doctor and called afterward to give us the report. Her heart was brand-new, and her leg was completely healed. She was a young pastor, and the devil had created all this illness in her life, but in a moment, God had removed it and made her as brand-new.

Healing from Demonic Attack

Once, I went to Taiwan to minister for a month, and we held big conventions where there were interpreters. One night, a woman came into the church with her two-year-old daughter in a stroller. The child could not hold her head up, and she was small for her age. An angel of the Lord was there, and he showed me a vision of this child. I don't want to disturb any who are mothers with what I say next. This may be difficult to receive, but it is important to be aware of the attacks that the enemy may wage against children. In this vision, I saw a small black serpent wrapped around that child's neck. I could see it as if I were looking at a television screen.

They brought the child up to the front row in a stroller, and the mother was sitting there praising God. The Holy Spirit said to me, *They won't be able to interpret what I'm saying. I want you to go down and lay hands on that baby.* So, I told the man there, and I went down and laid hands on the child and prayed and touched her neck. In the Spirit, I saw an angel of the Lord pull that snake off. When he did, the child's head was flopping. Then, the Lord said, *Now you must pray for strength in the neck.* The child had had this problem since birth, and she was now two years old. He said, *I will strengthen that baby's neck and head.* I prayed and prayed for the child and anointed her with oil. Before the service was over, the mother began jumping up and shouting because she noticed that the child began to look better and had started to be able to hold her little head up.

Backs Restored

These miracles just thrill my soul. I have seen all kinds of healings, including the healing of many back problems. I have prayed for people whose legs have grown out two or three inches. One man had not bent over in twenty years. We prayed, and Jesus healed his back.

A man named Ed wrote to me,

You prayed for my lower back, and yesterday and today I have been almost 100 percent pain free. I have been healed with the blood of Jesus. I swam in the pool today and had a great day. I praised Him all day and thanked Him for blessing me and healing my back.

Bishop [George] Bloomer gives the following account of when his mother was healed of severe back pain after doubting God's healing power.

"I was introduced to healing by my mother. Well-known faith healers of the twentieth century, such as Oral Roberts, A. A. Allen, and Kathryn Kuhlman, had a great influence on her. She had pictures and magazine and newspaper clippings about their services, which she cherished.

"Yet before this, for quite some time, she had suffered from a bad back condition. Though it's not clear to me where or when she was injured, I know that when I was growing up, she had excruciating pain and complained of her back hurting all the time.

"One evening, when I came home, she was sitting in front of the television, crying. I asked her what was wrong, and she told me that her back was on fire. 'Ma,' I asked, 'are you hurting? Do we need to call the doctor?' She began to explain, 'No. This is a good fire. It's like liniment.' Liniment was an awful, minty-smelling ointment that people used to rub on their backs and muscles to alleviate pain—similar to Aspercreme today. She continued, 'I feel like a heating pad is pressed against my spine, and it feels so good.' Then, pointing at the television screen, she said, 'I think that lady right there—look at her, George—has healed me.' I looked, and 'that lady' to whom my mother was referring was Kathryn Kuhlman.

"I was really amazed by my mother's statement because she had previously spent so much time trying to disprove miraculous healings, saying that they were something of the past. She would even thumb her nose at modern medicines and instead resort to using alternative treatments, such as herbs and exercises, to alleviate her pain, though to no avail. On that wonderful Saturday night, however, my mother received her healing, her miracle. Had it been any other night, my mother probably would not have seen Kathryn Kuhlman. You see, my mother was a Seventh-day Adventist, and they keep the Sabbath on Saturday. Had it been any other day, she would not have been watching Christian television. Had it been any other night, Kathryn Kuhlman would not have been on television, but God used her as a vessel to heal my mother. He did not use Kathryn Kuhlman simply for the physical healing of my mother's chronic pain, but more important, to reveal Himself to her in the Person of the Lord Jesus Christ.

"I, too, would go on to experience healings. Many times in my life, I have seen God's miraculous healing power. When I was a youth, I was strung out on drugs, and my heart actually stopped one night from a near-fatal drug overdose. Except by the grace of God, and through my mother's prayers, I would have died in the emergency room. But God had other plans for my life. God is real, and His power is evident."

Raised from the Dead!

Yes, God raises the dead, even in our day. I was preaching at a service in Illinois some years ago, and there was a woman sitting in the front row looking as stiff as a board. God revealed to me that she'd just died, so I went to her husband and whispered, "I think your wife has died." He replied, "Oh, she always looks like that." Even under the circumstances, it was funny to hear him say that, but I still insisted, "No, she's dead. God just revealed to me that she has died." So, we called 9-1-1, and when the paramedics came, she did not have a pulse. They placed her on a gurney, and, as they were rolling her out, she sat up. I looked over at her husband, who again said, "I told you, she always looks like that." In my heart, I knew that God had raised her from the dead. We later found out that she was diabetic and had taken too much insulin before the service and overdosed on it.

I have learned that when God is revealing something to me, I must have faith and obey because someone's life could depend upon how I react.

Another time, I was at my mother-in-law's church and was sitting beside an elderly woman whose nephew was preaching. She suddenly began sliding down in the chair. *Oh no*, I thought to myself. *If this woman dies in my mother-in-law's church, everyone is going to talk about it.* She just kept stiffening up and sliding down in the chair. I tried whispering to her nephew, but he couldn't hear me. Finally, I yelled up to the pulpit, "Your aunt has died!"

He jumped down and began giving her mouth-to-mouth resuscitation. When he did that, the most foul odor filled the entire sanctuary. It was unlike any smell I had ever experienced before. While we were waiting for the paramedics to come, I said to her nephew and my mother-in-law, "We have to pray for God to raise this woman from the dead because surely she is not ready to go meet the Lord!"

When the paramedics arrived, they couldn't get a pulse. As they were putting her on the gurney, I just could not let go of the fact that this woman, although she was ninety-something years old, was not ready to meet the Lord. I insisted, "Her soul is not right with God. We've got to remit her sins and give her life to God." So we continued to pray, and as they were rolling her out on the gurney, her hand moved. I rushed over to her and immediately asked, "Are you saved? If not, you need to get saved right now and give your life to God." We went through the sinner's prayer with her, and she got off the gurney. She said to us, "Do you know what I saw when I died? My soul came out of my body and I floated across this room and watched all of you as you prayed for me and gave me mouth-to-mouth resuscitation. When you were praying to God for my soul to go back into my body, it's like I had no control over it. It just went right back into my body." This is proof of just one of the many things that God can do.

From the cradle to the grave, God is with us. Whether you believe it or not, sometimes people lying on their deathbeds are those to whom God's grace is being extended because He wants to give them time to get their lives right with Him. We have to learn to take dominion over death. When we pray in the Holy Spirit, He knows the perfect prayer for us to pray over a dying person.

You have to have faith in whatever area of ministry God calls you to because it is meant to serve the needs of others.

The manifestation of the Spirit is given to each one for the profit of all: for to one is given the word of wisdom through the Spirit, to another the word of knowledge through the same Spirit, to another faith by the same Spirit, to another gifts of healings by the same Spirit, to another the working of miracles. (1 Corinthians 12:7–10 NKJV)

If you have cancer or some other ailment that is terminal, you must begin to claim a miracle, regardless of what it looks like in the natural. One time, when I was traveling overseas, I became very sick. I was so weak that I could barely move. I immediately began rebuking the devil because he was trying to fill my mind with all types of evil reports when I hadn't even been to the doctor to get a diagnosis. When you begin to curse the works of darkness, angels begin to work.

I made up my mind that I was going to the doctor. The doctors gave me an MRI and could not find anything wrong with me. Still, I was still so sick that I could barely hold up my head. Six weeks went by. Then, one night, I had a dream in which I saw Jesus on the cross. I saw Him being pierced in the side, and then He spoke to me in the dream and said, "By My stripes, you are healed." He began to explain to me, "Child, you have a fungus in your lungs, and you have to curse it in My name and I will heal you." So, I began doing that in the dream. I cursed the sickness in Jesus' name and put my trust in Him to heal me. I awoke the next morning with energy that I had not experienced in a very long time. All the weakness was completely gone!

Questions About Physical Healing

Many people have questions about physical healing when they deal with sickness and disease, and to conclude this chapter, I would like to address some of these concerns.

1. Should we use doctors and medicine, or should we just pray?

I believe that God does work in conjunction with doctors. There are many Holy Spirit-filled doctors and nurses today. Luke, the author of the gospel of Luke and the book of Acts, was a physician. In addition, many lives have been saved through medicine. People who don't know the Lord go to doctors and are healed of a number of ailments. Most of us who know the Lord have benefited from medical treatment, as well. We have to use the practical sense God has given us.

Yet I always put my trust in God when I have a physical need. I really believe that God is the main healer. *"I am the LORD who heals you"* (Exodus 15:26 NKJV). For example, I went to a Christian physician, and he discovered that I had a heart blockage. We prayed, and God healed me of this blockage. Other people with bad hearts have been healed in my meetings since this happened.

2. Are people healed in only a certain way?

One thing I have learned through my ministry travels and seeing God work in people's lives is never to second-guess God. Just when you think you have Him figured out or that He no longer performs the miraculous, He shows forth a great work.

We must be open to the various ways in which God may work. He loves us, and He wants us to know the depth of His concern for our well-being. Sometimes, we become so complacent in our conditions that we cease to call on the name of the Lord to help us.

Years ago, while I was in prayer, I had a vision of the Lord's banquet table. At the end of the table sat an outline of the Lord. There were hundreds of places set at the table, but only two seats were occupied. All the other seats were empty. The Lord asked me, "Where are the rest of them?"

"What, Lord?" I asked.

"Come and dine at the Master's table," was His only reply.

Then He began reminding me of a previous vision that He had shown me. In the middle of the night, I had dreamed of my kitchen—but it was a very elegant and spectacular version of the kitchen. In the natural, I had none of the things that filled this kitchen. But the kitchen had a set table that was fit for a king.

I had this dream night after night. And the Lord would say, "Come and dine at the Master's table. Come and dine." As I sat at the table, I kept noticing the empty chairs. Within what seemed like a two-hour period, only about ten people had joined the Lord at His table. As they came to the table, the Lord would speak to them and give them direction. The main point that I remember the Lord conveying was that we are to carry out the individual instructions that He has given to each of us. In other words, we have to throw off traditional ways of doing things. Any tradition that keeps us from seeking God with our whole hearts and entering into His presence is a hindrance. The religious leaders who rebuked Jesus for healing on the Sabbath were hindered by their self-imposed traditions. (See, for example, Luke 13:10–16.) We should not limit ourselves when it comes to seeking God and receiving from Him. Again, He may come when we least expect it and in a way that we hadn't thought He would show up in our lives.

In addition, at this table, God admonished all of us to walk in the shoes that He'd placed on our feet and not try to copy someone else's anointing. For instance, one person might have faith that God will heal him through the laying on of hands, while another might believe that God will heal her through the "miracle" of modern medicine. Whatever you do in life, do it in proportion to your faith. (See Romans 12:6–8.) In addition, don't put limits on God as He leads you. *"If you have faith as a mustard seed, you will say to this mountain, 'Move from here to there,' and it will move; and nothing will be impossible for you"* (Matthew 17:20 NKJV).

God can heal in many different ways. When He healed the blind man, for instance, Jesus spat on the ground and used clay to anoint the man's eyes. (See John 9:1–7.) Can you imagine someone today spitting on the ground and then using the dirt to anoint your eyes? Your first instinct might be to back away. However, we must realize that God sometimes heals in an unusual way in order to shock the normal thinking of humankind and to focus their attention on Him as Healer. Healing, then, sometimes causes quite a commotion.

> He [Jesus] *said to him* [the blind man], *"Go, wash in the pool of Siloam" (which is translated, Sent). So he went and washed, and came back seeing. Therefore the neighbors and those who previously had seen that he was blind said, "Is not this he who sat and begged?" Some said, "This is he." Others said, "He is like him." He said, "I am he."* (John 9:7–9 NKJV)

I believe that when the formerly blind man said, *"I am he"* (verse 9 NKJV), it was because he wanted to leave nothing to speculation. He was making it clear that he once had been blind but now was able to see by the miraculous workings of God.

Again, throughout my travels, I often see God healing people through means that do not always coincide with our earthly ways of thinking. Sometimes, I actually see angels standing beside the pastor of a church as he or she prays for somebody. I can see the Word of God coming out of the pastor's mouth like a sword. As the person who is being prayed for is anointed with oil, the sword goes into that person and cuts out that dark spot from the sick individual's body.

Some people may feel heat on their bodies when they're being healed because God is touching them. They actually feel the witness and the warmth of the power of God. That is also why it is so important for us to believe God. Can you imagine how many more could have been healed at the same time the blind man was healed if they had only believed? Instead, the Pharisees and others wasted time doubting Jesus and calling Him a sinner when they should have been believing Him for a miracle!

People often ask me how to get the healing anointing of God. It's no big secret! Remain persistent in prayer and continue to seek the face of God. For hours, I have sought God, kneeled before His presence, and allowed Him to speak to me through dreams and visions. There are many things we could do for the Lord if we'd just take the time to seek Him and listen to what He has to say. For instance, there have been times when I have visited convalescent homes where some of the elderly patients were so ill that they had slipped into comas. Whether it was time for them to be healed or to go home to be with the Lord, I still prayed for them as if they could hear, because I knew that their spirits could hear my prayers.

I went to one rest home where the same preachers had been going for about ten years. I asked these preachers, "Why don't you lead these elderly people to the Lord?"

They answered, "They can't hear you."

"We must believe God and pray for them," I replied.

As we prayed for them, tears began to stream down the faces of those elderly people who were in a comatose state, and we led them to the Lord. Don't ever put limitations on God. *"For now we see in a mirror, dimly"* (1 Corinthians 13:12 NKJV), but the more we come to know God, our understanding becomes enlightened. Unfortunately, because our conventional ways of thinking do not line up with God's supernatural manifestation, we unknowingly bind the Hand that holds the power to heal. Just remember, if God could raise Lazarus from the dead, surely He can heal us from sicknesses and diseases. Healing is a commission by God. He confirmed this fact when He sent the disciples out to preach with a purpose: *"And as you go, preach, saying, 'The kingdom of heaven is at hand.' Heal the sick, cleanse the lepers, raise the dead, cast out demons. Freely you have received, freely give"* (Matthew 10:7–8 NKJV).

A misconception regarding healing is that God always saves people first and then heals them, but He also heals people to demonstrate His power in order to save them and others. The miraculous works of God speak for themselves, which is why Jesus said, *"Believe Me for the sake of the works themselves"* (John 14:11 NKJV).

How many times might you have been in the presence of God when He was ready to heal and not known it? How many times have you traded the opportunity to receive a miracle for the hindrances that continue to stand between you and God? If you actually knew the answer to these questions, you might be dismayed.

God visits us often, but we fail to acknowledge His presence because we have been taught that He can show up only in a certain way or at a certain place. What if a beggar sat down beside you and said, "God sent me to lay hands on you to heal you"? Would you become turned off by this person's outward appearance and back away, or would you be able to sense the presence of God and receive the miracle God sent you that day? These are all very difficult questions, but ones that must be answered if we intend to ready ourselves for God's work in our lives. Whatever ails you is of great importance to God. He said in John 10:10 (nkjv) that He came that we might have life *"more abundantly."* God wants to exceed your expectations and pour out a blessing that you will not have room to receive. (See Malachi 3:10.) He wants to heal you, bless you, and enable you to go out and lay hands on others and see them recover from their sicknesses. (See Mark 16:18.)

3. What is the reason some people are not healed?

The question many ask is, "Why do some people who have faith in God for healing remain sick or even die instead of being healed, as others are who seem to have the same faith?"

We don't know. There are many mysteries that we do not understand. We're not God, and we don't have all the answers. Ultimately, God has control over our destinies when it comes to living or dying.

Rather than focus on what might not be happening in regard to healing, it is better to emphasize the power and authority that God has made available to us to receive healing. In the Word of God, we see that some people tried to interpret God's thinking. They wasted time blaming people's illnesses on sin, or on their parents' sins, rather than seeking a God-given cure for them.

In John 9, Jesus' disciples asked Him about the blind man, *"'Rabbi, who sinned, this man or his parents, that he was born blind?' Jesus answered, 'Neither this man nor his parents sinned, but that the works of God should be revealed in him'"* (John 9:2–3 nkjv). Jesus went on to explain that His job was to work the works of the One who sent Him. (See John 9:4 nkjv.) We might interpret this statement to mean that Jesus did not want to become bogged down with triviality. He had more important things to do, which were to heal the sick, raise the dead, and be the sacrifice for the sins of the world.

Whether we bring illness upon ourselves through bad eating habits, or whether illness just attacks us inexplicably, when we are sick, the only thing we want to know is, *How can I become healed from this ailment?* People who are sick or dying don't want to discuss whether they are sick because their parents have sinned. Instead, they seek God's mercy and relief. By equipping ourselves with the proper biblical knowledge concerning healing, we become better able to assist not only ourselves but also others who are in need.

None of us knows our appointed time to go home to be with the Lord. *"To everything there is a season, a time for every purpose under heaven: a time to be born, and a time to die...a time to kill, and a time to heal"* (Ecclesiastes 3:1–3 NKJV). Although we have seen that there are times when God raises people from the dead, there are other times when, no matter how hard we pray, the person we pray for is not raised up in this life.

This does not mean, however, that we should not pray for complete healing. God encourages us to pray and to seek His face, not only to understand His will, but also to receive the desires of our hearts: *"Delight yourself also in the LORD, and He shall give you the desires of your heart"* (Psalm 37:4 NKJV).

Likewise, sometimes God heals instantly, and sometimes He heals through a process. I had a heart blockage for two years before it was healed. I don't have all the answers, and I really don't know why God didn't heal it in the beginning. I think that is God's business. We know that by His stripes, we are healed. We see miracles, such as those shared in this book. So, I have truly learned to trust the Lord with everything. I've learned to lean on Him. I believe He's right on time.

4. Do people's sins cause their sicknesses?

Jesus said to the invalid whom He healed at the pool of Bethesda, *"See, you have been made well. Sin no more, lest a worse thing come upon you"* (John 5:14 NKJV). There are times when sin will cause sickness or other forms of trouble in life. Sickness and death in general are a result of sin. (See Romans 5:12–14.) In the Old Testament, God sometimes used sickness to punish the Israelites for their disobedience and to draw them back to Him. (See Numbers 21:5–9.) However, we must be careful not to pronounce that a certain illness was caused by specific sins. We must also realize that those who are sick do not always remain that way due to sin. One of the greatest misconceptions concerning healing is that those in need of a miracle might somehow have brought illness upon themselves. Again, as indicated in John 9, this is not always the case:

Now as Jesus passed by, He saw a man who was blind from birth. And His disciples asked Him, saying, "Rabbi, who sinned, this man or his parents, that he was born blind?" Jesus answered, "Neither this man nor his parents sinned, but that the works of God should be revealed in him."

(John 9:1–3 NKJV)

The disciples were focusing on sin when, instead, they should have been focusing on the opportunity for onlookers to witness the miraculous power of God.

A related question that is often asked is, *Why do bad things happen to good people?* The Word of the Lord declares that in this life, we will all go through trials and tribulations, but that God is faithful to deliver us from them all. *"In the world you will have tribulation; but be of good cheer, I have overcome the world"* (John 16:33 NKJV). Since Jesus has overcome and resides in us, then we, too, have the power to overcome "the world," including sickness and disease.

Journey into Word & Spirit

1. Is there some reason for which you think Jesus would not heal you?

2. Is there something the Lord is asking you to do, or someone you need to forgive (perhaps yourself), before you can receive God's healing?

Chapter excerpted from Mary K. Baxter, *A Divine Revelation of Healing* (New Kensington, PA: Whitaker House, 2009), chapter 6, "Healing for the Body."

About the Author

From the headquarters of her ministry, Divine Revelation, Inc., in Florida, evangelist Mary K. Baxter travels the world telling of her revelatory visits from the Lord. She has authored a number of books, including *A Divine*

Revelation of Hell, A Divine Revelation of Heaven, A Divine Revelation of the Spirit Realm, A Divine Revelation of Angels, A Divine Revelation of Spiritual Warfare, A Divine Revelation of Deliverance, A Divine Revelation of Prayer, and *The Power of the Blood.*

QUESTIONS AND ANSWERS
ON DIVINE HEALING

Maria Woodworth-Etter

6

QUESTIONS AND ANSWERS ON DIVINE HEALING

Maria Woodworth-Etter

Q. What is divine healing?

A. Divine healing is the act of God's grace, by the direct power of the Holy Spirit, by which the physical body is delivered from sickness and disease and restored to soundness and health.

Q. Have we any promise in the Bible that divine healing was ever intended to be an attainable blessing to the people of God?

A. Yes. There are many such promises. We find it given to the people of Israel in a special covenant promise. *"If thou wilt diligently hearken to the voice of the LORD thy God, and wilt do that which is right in his sight, and wilt give ear to his commandments, and keep all His statutes, I will put none of these diseases upon thee, which I have brought upon the Egyptians: for I am the LORD that healeth thee"* (Exodus 15:26). *"And ye shall serve the LORD your God, and* *he shall bless thy bread and thy water; and I will take sickness away from the midst of thee"* (Exodus 23:25).

Q. Does the Bible prove that any of the people of God ever enjoyed this blessing?

A. Yes. We read that even before this covenant blessing was promised, the physical condition of the people was perfect, which indicates plainly that God had a special interest in their health. There were at least two and one-half million people in the Exodus from Egypt, *"and there was not one feeble person among their tribes"* (Psalm 105:37). Moses enjoyed this blessing in a special manner. (See Deuteronomy 34:7.) So also did Caleb in an unusual experience of preservation and health to an old age. (See Joshua 14:10–11.) David personally knew of the benefits and blessings of healing. (See Psalm 6:2; 30:2; 103:1–4.) Whenever Israel lived up to the covenant conditions, they all had the benefits of healing and health. (See Psalm 107:20; 2 Chronicles 30:20.) Hezekiah had a personal experience of the same. (See 2 Kings 20:1–5.)

Q. Was this blessing ever promised to anyone else than the Jews?

A. Yes. It is given in prophecy as a redemption blessing, which, together with all other gospel blessings through Christ, is offered to both Jew and Gentile. (See Galatians 3:27–29.)

Q. What does prophecy say about divine healing?

A. There is more said about it in prophecy than we have time at present to read, but I will just quote a few verses, and the rest can be read at your leisure. *"Then the eyes of the blind shall be opened, and the ears of the deaf shall be unstopped. Then shall the lame man leap as an hart, and the tongue of the dumb sing"* (Isaiah 35:5–6). This very prophecy is referred to by Jesus Himself in Matthew 11:5–6, where it was daily being fulfilled, *"The blind receive their sight, and the lame walk, the lepers are cleansed, and the deaf hear, the dead are raised up, and the poor have the gospel preached to them."* Another very plain prophecy is found in Isaiah 53:4: *"Surely he hath borne our griefs, and carried our sorrows."* The fulfillment of this wonderful voice of inspiration is found in Matthew 8:17: *"Himself took our infirmities, and bare our sicknesses."* It is admitted by all reliable translators and the most eminent Hebrew scholars, such as Barnes, Magee, Young, and Leeser, that Isaiah 53:4 in its literal rendering corresponds exactly with Matthew 8:17. We see, therefore, that the latter is a direct reference to the former. Then the beautiful prophecy of salvation and healing is found in the following verse, Isaiah 53:5: *"But he was wounded for our transgressions, he was bruised for our iniquities: the chastisement of our peace was upon him; and with his stripes we are healed."* These prophecies all point to the redemption work of Jesus, which finds its center in the cross. The apostle Peter refers to this verse just quoted in the following language: *"Who his own self bare our sins in his own body on the tree, that we, being dead to sins, should live unto righteousness: by whose stripes ye were healed"* (1 Peter 2:24). The following references will enable you to see that more is said in prophecy about healing: Isaiah 42:7; Isaiah 61:1, fulfilled in Luke 4:18–21; prophecy in Malachi 4:2, fulfilled in Matthew 4:16; Luke 1:78–79. These are all fulfilled in redemption.

Q. Do you believe that the Bible teaches divine healing as a redemption blessing?

A. Yes. Do you not see how plain this is made in the prophecies just quoted and in their fulfillment? Jesus worked in every respect, in His life, ministry, death, and resurrection, just according to the redemption plan. His words and deeds are the divine expression of this redemption plan, and we can clearly see that healing for the body is placed upon an equality with healing for the soul. Both are obtained upon the same grounds, obedience and faith.

Q. Can a person possess salvation without healing?

A. Yes, he may. While both are obtained by faith, yet they may not both be obtained by the same act of faith. Jesus will be to us just what our faith takes Him for.

Q. Did Jesus heal everybody?

A. Yes, all who came to Him in faith. Read Matthew 4:23–24 and Matthew 12–15.

Q. But they did not seem to have faith, did they?

A. Yes. If you read the references just mentioned, you will notice the people came to Him for healing and followed Him. At Nazareth, His own town, where He had been brought up, He could do no great work among them, *"because of their unbelief"* (Matthew 13:58). At Capernaum, where some of the most remarkable healings were wrought, the people were a believing people. Out of nineteen of the most prominent individual cases of healing in the ministry of Christ and the apostles, there are twelve of these where their faith is spoken of. The rest are mentioned sufficiently plain to show that faith brought the healing in every case.

Q. Did not Jesus heal arbitrarily, for the sole purpose of establishing His divinity?

A. No. He healed according to the law of redemption and because of His great compassion for suffering humanity. (Matthew 14:14.)

Q. Didn't divine healing cease when Jesus finished His earthly ministry?

A. No. It was more wonderfully manifested in the ministry of the apostles after the Day of Pentecost. See Acts 5:12–16; 3:1–16; 14:8–10; 9:17–18; 8:6–8; 19:11–12; 14:19–20; 9:33–35; 36:42; 20:8–12; 28:3–6, 8. This proves clearly that divine healing is a redemption blessing for the entire Holy Spirit dispensation.

Q. But we are taught that it was only for the beginning of the gospel dispensation. How about that?

A. The Bible does not teach any such doctrine.

Q. But it does teach that *"when that which is perfect is come, then that which is in part shall be done away"* (1 Corinthians 13:10). How about this?

A. This Scripture has no reference to divine healing or any of the redemption blessings, that they shall be done away with in this dispensation. If there ever has been a time in this dispensation when it could have been said with reference to the full possession and manifestation of the gospel blessings, that *"that which is perfect is come,"* it was when the Holy Spirit came at Pentecost. But after this we see mighty works of salvation and healing, and they were in no sense done away with, but were greatly increased. So you see the "done away with" argument has no scriptural basis whatever. As long as the dispensation of grace shall last, so long shall the benefits of grace be extended to *"whosoever will"* (Revelation 22:17).

Q. Well, then, when was divine healing done away?

A. In the design of God it was never done away.

Q. Do you mean to say that it was perpetuated in the primitive church?

A. Certainly it was. History shows that for several centuries there was no other means of healing practiced in the church.

Q. But what after that?

A. Just what crowded out all other gospel truths—the superstitions and unbelief of the apostasy. But, thank God, the darkness is past and *"the Sun of righteousness...with healing in his wings"* (Malachi 4:2) is shining salvation and health to all who will forsake all their old doctrines, creeds, and superstitions and get back upon the old apostolic foundation, the Word of God.

Q. But how may I know that it is still God's will to heal?

A. Just as you may know that it is His will to save—by His Word. His Word is His will.

Q. But it may be His will not to heal me.

A. You must go outside of God's Word to find standing ground for such a conclusion, for there is nothing inside of the Bible about healing but what corresponds with our blessed text: *"Himself took our infirmities, and bare our sicknesses."* Most people who argue that it might not be God's will to heal them are at the same time taking medicine and employing every possible human agency to get well. Why be so inconsistent? Why fight against God's will? If it is His will for you not to get well, then die. Stop fighting against God.

Q. But doesn't sickness come from God as a blessing?

A. No. It never comes from God except in a permissive sense, the same as a temptation comes to us; and sickness is never a blessing to us except as any other temptation or trial may be considered a blessing. The blessing is in the deliverance and healing. Every person who has ever experienced the healing touch of God knows what a blessing to the soul comes with it. Sickness is an abnormal condition of the body and cannot be a blessing from God.

Q. If it does not come from God, then where does it come from?

A. It comes from the devil and was always dealt with by Jesus in His earthly ministry as a work of the devil. The Word of God plainly teaches us that the devil is the author of disease. Read John 2:7; Luke 3:16; Acts 1:38.

Q. But aren't there some other Scriptures that teach us that sickness comes from God?

A. Only in a permissive sense.

Q. Does the Bible teach us that God intends to be the Healer of His people without the use of medicine?

A. Yes. It nowhere commands the use of medicine with prayer and faith.

Q. But how about Hezekiah's figs, the blind man's clay, and Timothy's wine?

A. It is true Isaiah told Hezekiah to take a lump of figs, but this has nothing to do with the New Testament means of healing. Also it is very evident that the figs did not heal him; but God said, *"I will heal thee"* (2 Kings 20:5). Jesus did not use the clay on the eyes of the blind man for any curative power, for He commanded the man at once to go and wash it off. No one has heard of blindness from birth being healed by the use of clay as a medicine before or since then. It is evident that the spittle and clay were used by Jesus as a requirement of submission and obedience from the blind man. The thought must have been repulsive and humiliating to him as the clay was applied to his eyes, but, like Naaman, he submitted and obeyed and received the blessing unspeakable of healing. Wine was recommended to Timothy as an article of diet and would not be objectionable today, in its proper use, under similar circumstances.

Q. Aren't medicines recognized in the Word of God?

A. Yes. Let us read how it recognizes them. *"Thou hast no healing medicines"* (Jeremiah 30:13). *"In vain shalt thou use many medicines"* (Jeremiah 46:11). *"A merry heart doeth good like a medicine* [margin, *to a medicine*, showing that the merry heart is better than the medicine]" (Proverbs 17:22). *"And the fruit thereof shall be for meat, and the leaf thereof for medicine"* (Ezekiel 47:12). This latter reference does not mean any material remedy but is prophetic of the Tree of Life and divine healing. (See Revelation 22:2.) Thus we see the Word of God places no intrinsic value upon medicine.

Q. Is not the ministry of physicians for the body designed of God, the same as the ministry of the Gospel for the soul?

A. No. The greater portion of the physicians of the land are ungodly people; many of them are professed infidels and were never designed of God to administer drugs and poisons to anyone, much less to the people of God, whose bodies are the sacred temples of the Holy Spirit. The true ministers of the Gospel are the ministers for soul and body. *"And they departed, and went through the towns, preaching the gospel, and healing every where"* (Luke 9:6). *"And they went forth, and preached everywhere, the Lord working with them, and confirming the word with signs following"* (Mark 16:20).

Q. But is not the ministry of physicians recognized in the Bible?

A. Yes. Let us read how it recognizes them. *"But ye are forgers of lies, ye are all physicians of no value"* (Job 13:4). *"And Asa in the thirty and ninth year of his reign was diseased in his feet, until his disease was exceeding great: yet in his disease he sought not to the LORD, but to the physicians"* (2 Chronicles 16:12). *"And had suffered many things of many physicians, and had spent all that she had, and was nothing bettered, but rather grew worse"* (Mark 5:26). These Scriptures show that the Bible gives no very favorable recognition of physicians.

Q. Wasn't anointing with oil the mode of doctoring in Bible times?

A. No. While some kinds of oil may have some medical value for some kinds of diseases, it was not at all designed for any such use in connection with the prayer of faith in healing the sick. If anointing was the mode of doctoring, the church would have had no need of instruction in this respect, for it would have been a common practice everywhere by the doctors. Had this been the mind of the apostle, then he would have assigned the work of anointing to the doctors. "Elders are not masseurs."

Journey into Word & Spirit

1. What thoughts have kept you from believing that God desires to heal you? Write them down and then go back through this chapter and/or your own Bible to find specific Scriptures that combat those doubts.

2. Based on this chapter, how can you be sure that God desires to heal you?

3. Play some worship music and spend some time in prayer. Imagine that Jesus is with you and ask Him to speak a word directly to your heart.

Chapter excerpted from Maria Woodworth-Etter, *Signs and Wonders* (New Kensington, PA: Whitaker House, 1997), 184–189.

About the Author

Often described as the "Grandmother of the Pentecostal Movement," Maria Woodworth-Etter was a figurehead of the early Pentecostal and charismatic Christian movement.

Born in 1844 in Lisbon, Ohio, she had a ministry that touched hundreds of thousands of people, and through the power of her books, even millions. Thousands of sick, lame, possessed, and lost people attended her Holy Spirit-filled meetings, and many were healed.

WHY SOME PEOPLE ARE NOT HEALED

Randy Clark

7

WHY SOME PEOPLE ARE NOT HEALED

Randy Clark

Some people seem to have an extreme amount of faith, and they are not healed. Some say the person must have unconfessed sin in their life; but, for most, they are dealing with everything that they can, and they are not healed. It puts a burden of guilt and condemnation on them that they shouldn't have to carry. I don't know the real answer for why people aren't healed, or why they lose their healing. Sometimes, the prayer team didn't deal with the root, and it grew a new fruit. Sometimes, it's an afflicting spirit, and we didn't tell them that they have authority and power and can speak to it and tell it to leave and maintain your healing. Or they move into unbelief....

Why are some people healed or not healed? I don't know. There is something about sovereignty that I don't understand. I do know that those who believe healing is in the atonement see many more people healed when they pray.

There is a direct connection between the ways of God related to salvation and related to healing. Not everyone who hears the message of salvation gets saved. Not everyone who hears the message of healing gets healed. Not everyone who appears to have been saved, based upon the fruit later, really did get saved. Not everybody that thought they were healed in the moment, three or four days later, really were healed or maintained healing. We don't always understand why.

God never said I had to understand it to do it, to pray for it, to believe in it. If my faith is waiting upon my understanding, I'm never going to go very far.

I tell our people in our teams that we are training two things I never want them to do [are] to tell people they didn't get healed because they didn't have enough faith or [tell them] that they didn't get healed because they have sin in their lives, because those are judgments; those are accusations. You're lining up with Satan, the accuser of the brethren, rather than the Holy Spirit, who is to help us. Even if you think this person needs more faith, you never judge them; you encourage them, and you try to do things with them and come along beside them and strengthen their faith.

Journey into Word & Spirit

1. Are there any judgments people have spoken about you that have caused you to falter in your belief that God can heal you? What were they?

2. Write a prayer of forgiveness and blessing for those who have hurt you.

3. Spend some time with the Lord and ask Him to heal the wounds of judgment and accusation that others have committed against you. Then, renew your faith in God's love for you and in His desire to heal you.

Chapter based on Randy Clark's video teaching "When Healing Doesn't Happen," http://www.xpmedia.com/video/1882/when-healing-doesnt-happen.

About the Author

Randy Clark is the founder of Global Awakening, a teaching, healing, and impartation ministry that seeks to "train, equip, and mobilize people of all ages, nationalities, and backgrounds to reproduce the supernatural work of the Holy Spirit…to fulfill the Great Commission." For more information, please visit https://www.healingcertification.com and https://globalawakening.com.

HEALTH AND SALVATION BY THE NAME OF JESUS

Andrew Murray

8

HEALTH AND SALVATION BY THE NAME OF JESUS

Andrew Murray

*"And his name through faith in his name hath made this man strong,
whom ye see and know: yea, the faith which is by him hath given him
this perfect soundness in the presence of you all."*
—Acts 3:16

*"Be it known unto you all, and to all the people of Israel, that by the
name of Jesus Christ of Nazareth, whom ye crucified, whom God
raised from the dead, even by him doth this man stand here before you
whole....Neither is there salvation in any other: for there is none other
name under heaven given among men, whereby we must be saved."*
—Acts 4:10, 12

After Pentecost, the paralytic was healed through Peter and John at the gate of the temple. It was *"in the name of Jesus Christ of*

Nazareth" that they said to him, *"Rise up and walk"* (Acts 3:6). As soon as the people in their amazement ran together to them, Peter declared that it was the name of Jesus that had so completely healed the man.

As a result of this miracle and of Peter's discourse, many people who had heard the Word believed. (See Acts 4:4.) The next day, Peter repeated these words before the Sanhedrin: *"By the name of Jesus Christ of Nazareth… doth this man stand here before you whole"*; and then he added, *"There is none other name under heaven…whereby we must be saved."* This statement of Peter declares to us that the name of Jesus both heals and saves. We have here a teaching of the highest importance for divine healing.

We see that healing and health form part of Christ's salvation. Peter clearly stated this in his discourse to the Sanhedrin when, having spoken of healing, he immediately went on to speak of salvation by Christ. In heaven, even our bodies will have their part in salvation. Salvation will not be complete for us until our bodies enjoy the full redemption of Christ. Shouldn't we believe in this work of redemption here below? Even here on earth, the health of our bodies is a fruit of the salvation that Jesus has acquired for us.

We also see that health, as well as salvation, is to be obtained by faith. The natural tendency of man by nature is to bring about his own salvation by his works, and it is only with difficulty that he comes to receive it by faith. But when it is a question of the healing of the body, he has still more difficulty in seizing it. He finally accepts salvation through Christ, because by no other means can he open the door of heaven. But it is much easier for him to accept well-known remedies for his body. Why, then, should he seek divine healing?

Happy is he who comes to understand that it is the will of God to heal, to manifest the power of Jesus, and to reveal to us His fatherly love. It is also His will that we exercise and confirm our faith, to make us prove the power of redemption in the body as well as in the soul. The body is part of our being. Even the body has been saved by Christ. Therefore, our Father wills to manifest the power of redemption in our bodies, and to let men see that Jesus lives. Oh, let us believe in the name of Jesus! Was it not in the name of Jesus that perfect health was given to the crippled man? And were not the words *"Thy faith hath made thee whole"* (Mark 5:34) pronounced when the woman with the issue of blood was healed? Let us seek, then, to obtain divine healing.

Wherever the Spirit acts with power, He works divine healings. If ever there was an abundance of miracles, it was at Pentecost, for then the word of the apostles worked mightily, and the pouring out of the Holy Spirit was great. Well, it is precisely because the Spirit acted powerfully that His working was so visible in the body. If divine healing is seen but rarely in our day, we can attribute it to no other cause than that the Spirit does not act with power. The unbelief of worldlings and the lack of zeal among believers stop His working. The healings that God is giving here and there are the initial signs of all the spiritual graces that are promised to us, and only the Holy Spirit reveals the almightiness of the name of Jesus to operate such healings. Let us pray earnestly for the Holy Spirit, let us place ourselves unreservedly under His direction, and let us seek to be firm in our faith in the name of Jesus, whether for preaching salvation or for the work of healing.

God grants healing to glorify the name of Jesus. Let us seek to be healed by Jesus so that His name may be glorified. It is sad to see how little the power of His name is recognized, how little it is used in preaching and prayer. Treasures of divine grace—of which Christians deprive themselves by their lack of faith and zeal—are hidden in the name of Jesus.

It is the will of God to glorify His Son in the church, and He will do it wherever He finds faith. Whether among believers or among the heathen, He is ready with virtue from on high to awaken consciences and to bring hearts to obedience. God is ready to manifest the power of His Son and to do it in striking ways in bodies as well as in souls. Let us believe it for ourselves, and let us believe it for others—for the circle of believers around us and also for the church in the whole world. Let us give ourselves to believe with firm faith in the power of the name of Jesus. Let us ask great things in His name, counting on His promise, and we will see that God still does wonders by the name of His holy Son.

Journey into Word & Spirit

1. What "treasure of divine grace" do you want to ask God for?

2. Write down what this chapter has enabled you to discover (or rediscover) about the power of the name of Jesus.

3. Spend some time with the Lord and ask Him to give you a vision of what your life will look like without illness or disease. Think about how you would feel if Jesus suddenly said to you, "I am the Lord who heals you. Be made whole," and you were instantly healed.

Chapter excerpted from Andrew Murray, *Divine Healing* (New Kensington, PA: Whitaker House, 1982), chapter 4, "Health and Salvation by the Name of Jesus."

About the Author

South African pastor and author Andrew Murray (1828–1917) was an amazingly prolific writer. Murray began writing on the Christian life for his congregation as an extension of his local pastoral work, but he became internationally known for his books, such as *With Christ in the School of Prayer* and *Abide in Christ*, that searched men's hearts and brought them into a deep relationship with Christ.

BE HEALED

Marilyn Hickey

9

BE HEALED

Marilyn Hickey

God's supernatural touch in the life of a Christian is His "dinner bell" to the world; it rings out the invitation, "Come and dine." (See Isaiah 55:1–3.) Yes, it is a blessing to the one who receives it, but it also affords that person the opportunity to be an undeniable testimony to the unbeliever. The world should see every one of us walking in divine health, divine prosperity, and divine power and authority. It would be impossible for me to count the times I've seen miraculous healings open the door of people's hearts; and they, too, have stepped into the kingdom to sit and to sup with Jesus and to taste the good things He has for them. (See Revelation 3:20.)

I'm thinking now of a woman who "sowed" a godly life before her unsaved husband. Miracles in her life had repeatedly rung the dinner bell, but the chimes had fallen on deaf ears. Years went by, and she had plenty of time to either give up or keep on sowing precious seeds for an even bigger harvest. Then, this man was stricken with a serious heart attack. Of course, the devil would like to have taken him out of the game before he reached "home." But do you know that God and His team are better at playing the game of life than the devil and his team are at playing the game of death?

This unbelieving husband was touched by the miraculous power of God in such a dramatic way that just a few days after the heart attack, the doctors were scratching their heads in wonder. Every test showed the man had a normal heart, as though he had never had a heart attack. Isn't that just like the Lord? In this case, God performed the healing on the unbeliever himself. The heart attack brought the man to attention, and the miracle he experienced in his own body finally caused him to give his attention to the gospel. He couldn't deny his own healing, and he knew Jesus Christ had a claim on his life. The wife not only saw her husband's physical heart healed, but she also saw his spirit touched by the power of God.

The ringing of God's dinner bell can be heard all over the earth. God does not show partiality; Jesus died for the whole world. (See Acts 10:34–35.) God's table is set for every kindred and every tribe (see Revelation 5:9), and they are coming by the thousands to His banquet. On one of my missions trips to Russia, my ministry team and I saw thousands respond to God's dinner bell as we witnessed miracle after miracle of healing. The anointing was so heavy that all the members of the team saw people healed as the team prayed for them.

After one of the meetings, a team member had just stepped outside the building when a Russian lady shoved her daughter in front of her. This lady had heard the dinner bell, and she was determined that her child would hear it, too. Although there was a language barrier, the mother was able to show the woman that her child was deaf. The woman prayed, and instantly the little girl's ears were opened—she could hear! One woman on our team was healed of terrible varicose veins in her legs after three other team members prayed for her. This woman, who spoke fluent Russian, received her miracle at a time when she was "feeding" the Word of God to a group of hungry Russians. Again, the dinner bell rang.

God orchestrated another miraculous situation on this trip to Russia. One man and his wife went with gifts and money for a Russian couple they had never met. Friends of theirs had loaded them with the gifts for the husband and wife. The two Russians traveled nine hundred miles to Moscow, where we were, to receive the gifts from America. The husband and wife were a captive audience in our meeting, and they both accepted Jesus as their

Savior and Lord. These precious people received the greatest healing of all, the healing of their souls. I share this story to illustrate how infinitely God cares for all of us. Now, this Russian family has the gift of salvation to share with their friends, and the gift just keeps on giving.

> *Every good gift and every perfect gift is from above, and comes down from the Father of lights, with whom there is no variation or shadow of turning.* (James 1:17 NKJV)

Every one of us in Christ has received the power to be like our heavenly Father. Since there is no change in Him, there should be no change in us, except to be continually changing into a more perfect likeness of Jesus:

> *But we all, with unveiled face, beholding as in a mirror the glory of the Lord, are being transformed into the same image from glory to glory, just as by the Spirit of the Lord.* (2 Corinthians 3:18 NKJV)

When we step on the rung of God's ladder marked "healing," the next step we take should be a step up to "health." You'll never progress upward if you take a step backward.

When we have received a healing, it is never God's intention for us to lose it. In the fullness of Christ's humanity, He demonstrated to us that we can continually walk in victory and health through the power of the Holy Spirit. Even though Jesus was tempted in every way we will ever be tempted (see Hebrews 2:1; 4:15–16), His earthly life was continual proof that we, too, can live constantly in the life of God. We don't have to be well today and sick tomorrow. We can be unchanging in the power of God's divine life.

Three Unique Aspects of God's Healing Power

Look with me at three things that are unique about God's healing power.

Geographical Location Cannot Hinder It

First, geographical location can't hinder the power of God to heal. Again, when Jesus healed the centurion's servant, the servant wasn't there with Him.

Jesus spoke the word, and the servant was healed. When Jesus spoke a word in Israel, a woman's daughter was healed in Phoenicia....Psalm 107:20...says that God sends His Word to heal. Every time we pray a healing prayer for someone who is not with us, the Word is being sent to heal. I might add that God's power to heal is not stronger in one place than it is in another, simply because of location. We tend to think everything is better in America, but I want to tell you that more people are being healed today in Third World nations than in the United States.

Jesus Always Knows the Outcome

Next, Jesus always knows the end from the beginning; He knows the outcome of every illness. Jesus didn't rush down to Bethany when He received news of Lazarus' critical illness. He waited in Jerusalem until He knew by the Holy Spirit that Lazarus was no longer ill but dead. This was a heartbreaking situation for Mary and Martha, but Jesus knew they soon would be rejoicing over a greater miracle than healing. Jesus raised their brother from the dead! (See John 11:1–45.) If we stay in God's Word until we are convinced of His promises, we don't have to get rattled and nervous about the end result of a difficult matter. We can know that God intends to bring healing and victory every time. That is always His purpose, and He has the power to bring it to pass for those who are trusting in Him.

Jesus' Healing Is Complete

The third unique thing about the Lord's healing is that it is complete. He doesn't do a halfway job. However, we sometimes receive healing for one thing in our bodies, while another physical problem seems to drag on endlessly. In some cases, it seems much easier to believe for the healing of "little" things, while "bigger" things seem beyond the reach of our faith. That is not the way the Lord wants it to be. In His earthly ministry, He made people whole; He didn't leave them partially well or well in one part of their bodies and sick in another part.

Jesus Still Heals Today

Even though there is a common notion in "parts" of the body of Christ that Jesus does not heal today, the Lord is still healing multitudes of people all around them. If human bodies were made completely whole by Jesus' touch, I'm certain that God doesn't want some of Christ's body well and some of His body sick. It is a tragic irony that there are "parts" of our Lord's body that remain in sickness because of ignorance and unbelief. The Lord Jesus wants to touch all believers and make them completely well.

Healing didn't die out with the apostles, as some believe. Note that many people who were healed in the New Testament were not healed by the apostles. Stephen and Philip, who were both deacons, performed great wonders and miracles among the people. (See Acts 6:8; 8:6–7.) A man in Damascus laid hands on Paul, and he regained his sight. (See Acts 9:10–19.) Remember also that Paul—who was not one of the original twelve apostles—healed numerous people, and he did not begin to heal until after Jesus had ascended to heaven. (See, for example, Acts 28:8–9.)

Peter declared that our healing was purchased by the stripes (wounds) that Jesus took upon Himself at Calvary. (See 1 Peter 2:24.) The finished work of Calvary stands forever; and if Jesus is the same yesterday, today, and forever, then you and I can still be healed by those stripes!

What Prevents Americans from Being Healed

I next want to examine some things that are keeping Americans from being healed or that cost us our healing after we have received it. Remember, God not only wants us to get it, but He also wants us to *keep* it! I'm going to deal strictly with those who live in America, because our whole society is being hurt and damaged by wrong thoughts, attitudes, and actions. I call this condition "American paganism." Pagans are irreligious or hedonistic (self-indulgent to the extreme) people. In general, Americans "do their own thing"; if it feels good, we do it—whether or not it hurts anyone else. Praise the Lord, we still have some "salty" Christians who are preserving our nation.

> *A sound heart is life to the body....Wisdom rests in the heart of him who has understanding, but what is in the heart of fools is made known. Righteousness exalts a nation, but sin is a reproach to any people.*
> (Proverbs 14:30, 33–34 NKJV)

The "Eat, Drink, and Be Merry, for Tomorrow We Die" Attitude

There is the attitude in our culture that you are young only once, so live it up BIG. It's the hopeless philosophy of the "eat, drink, and be merry, for tomorrow we die" crowd. (See Ecclesiastes 8:15.) Our highways have become "slaughterhouses" for the drunk driver. Americans spend billions of dollars on junk food. And tens of millions of people "play" on the Lord's Day instead of worshipping in His house.

Now, I want to bring this closer to home. Almost without realizing it, we Christians also are permeated with these attitudes. What about the quantities of junk food, carbonated drinks, and empty calories we consume? Or what about the "sipping saints"? Do we think that if it tastes good, we can put it in our bodies without paying the consequences? Christian bodies are not immune to sickness. What about the types of TV programs and movies we watch, or the books and magazines we read? What are you looking at on the Internet? Let me tell you, folks, if only junk goes in, only junk will come out. Let's feast on life and not on death! We receive only one body in which to live this life, and a body used for self-indulgence will surely not be full of health.

The Desire for Instant Gratification

Another attitude that has invaded American thought is that we must have instant gratification. We can't wait for anything. We want instant service, instant potatoes, instant coffee, and instant credit. We have drive-through windows at fast-food restaurants and banks, we have express lanes at the supermarket, and we have microwave ovens to heat our "prepared" foods. The list of our "modern conveniences" is endless, but we hardly think about it as we sail through life in the fast lane. Isn't all of this what we deserve?

Let's take a closer look at our "instant" society. Our nation is trillions of dollars in debt, a number of our politicians have been involved in various scandals, banks are going under, all manner of businesses are going bankrupt, and charge cards have plunged multitudes into incredible debt. And we are slaughtering the unborn, who are the future of our nation. Where is instant gratification taking us? I know we are not all living this way, and I certainly enjoy my modern conveniences; but the attitude that we must have everything we want at the moment we want it is thoughtless and foolish. It leads to heartache and failure; it leads to sickness and death, as we disregard the lives of others, overstress ourselves, and don't take proper care of our bodies, minds, and spirits.

The "Victim Complex"

Americans also have a bad habit of blaming someone or something else for every problem. We take no personal responsibility for our problems. It is always the fault of someone else. America has a "victim" complex. "I wouldn't be sick if this hadn't happened," or "I wouldn't have these problems if I had been loved as a child," or "I grew up in a poor home, my parents were divorced, and my teachers didn't understand me." Secular psychology and psychiatry feed these attitudes, but they don't often present positive solutions. Some lawyers encourage greedy people to sue for every possible cause—real or imagined—so their clients can get what they "deserve" and the lawyers can line their own pockets.

Do you know where all this began? It began with the fall of humanity in the garden of Eden. Adam blamed God for giving him Eve, and Eve blamed the serpent for deceiving her; but God held both Adam and Eve accountable for their sin problem. I realize that many people are damaged by the things that have happened to them, and my heart aches for hurting people. However, there is only one way out of the hurt and the pain. People must stop placing blame, accept responsibility for their lives and their futures, and give the past to Jesus. He is the Healer—the only One who can truly heal our minds, our emotions, and our bodies.

A Dismissal of Everything That Is Beyond Our Understanding

Another mark of American paganism is our insistence upon everything being logical to the human mind. We have become so intellectual that if we can't understand something, we won't believe it. When it isn't in the realm of the natural, where we can hear it, see it, smell it, feel it, or taste it, we simply refuse to believe. If it isn't explainable, we toss it out. This is ridiculous. If we wait to figure out everything, we are going to wait a long time. We are going to miss God, and we are going to miss miracles. Don't miss your miracle of healing because you don't understand how God does it.

How many doctors can explain the essence of life because they know the parts of the human body and how they function? Nevertheless, we still go to doctors. How many astronomers can explain what holds the world in place because they can chart the galaxies? However, the exact precision of the universe is miraculous! Can the evolutionist tell you the origin of that first enzyme or slime that he thinks began the process of life? Do theologians understand everything in the Bible? Of course not. Neither do you nor I; but I accept it as truth, enjoy its blessings, and daily expect the Lord to open my spiritual eyes to greater revelation of the truths in His living Book.

There is no mortal, no matter what his genius, who can begin to figure out the mind and ways of God. Even the least of God's thoughts are greater than any human thought or imagination, *"because the foolishness of God is wiser than men, and the weakness of God is stronger than men"* (1 Corinthians 1:25 NKJV). We know that God is never foolish or weak; but with this impossible comparison, we should see that His wisdom and power immeasurably transcend any human thought or strength. In spite of this fact, the Lord promises to put His wisdom and power to work on our behalf *"immeasurably more than all we ask or imagine"* (Ephesians 3:20 NIV).

When we place our trust and confidence in the Lord, He is able to lift us from the natural into the supernatural with one touch of His miraculous power. What difference does it make if we can't understand the operations of God? We can still enjoy all His benefits. The miracle of healing is one of those benefits. God has put into the human body the natural ability to heal itself of many sicknesses, so even without a supernatural miracle, your body is a miracle healing machine. Don't abuse it.

> *Let the wicked forsake his way, and the unrighteous man his thoughts; let him return to the LORD, and He will have mercy on him; and to our God, for He will abundantly pardon. "For My thoughts are not your thoughts, nor are your ways My ways," says the LORD. "For as the heavens are higher than the earth, so are My ways higher than your ways, and My thoughts than your thoughts."* (Isaiah 55:7–9 NKJV)

If we try to figure out everything, it is going to get us out of faith. I can't explain miracles; but when I need one, all that matters is whether I can receive it. I can't afford to lose faith; that is far worse than "losing face." There is no one who can explain how cancers disappear, discs are replaced in spines, or arms and legs are lengthened. No one can explain how a drug addict or an alcoholic is set free in an instant from those horrible bondages. Nevertheless, anyone who has ever received such a miracle doesn't question that it happened.

Once, I called upon a young man in our congregation to report the healing of his knees. I didn't ask him to tell the congregation how the miracle happened—I just asked him to share his testimony, and we all rejoiced with him. Now he could walk without pain and do many things he couldn't do before. This man didn't know how God had healed his knees; he just appreciated and enjoyed the benefits. During this time, I was teaching a series on healing in our church, and we saw miracle after miracle. I can't explain how eyes, ears, and backs were healed; I can't explain how tumors and warts vanished; but they did. Years ago, my back was healed when an evangelist prayed for me. One of my arms was longer than the other, but, when he prayed, my outstretched arms became the same length before my eyes, and I've never had the back problem since. It was an unexplainable miracle.

What Is Causing Americans to Be Sick

We've looked at some attitudes and actions that prevent Americans from being healed. Now, it is time to look more closely at some of the things that produce sickness in Americans and keep them that way.

Prepared Foods

One of the things that is making Americans sick is our "supermarket diet"—a diet that is full of prepared foods. Nutritionists warn us not to eat the contents of a package if we can't pronounce the ingredients on the label. Much of what we take from the supermarket shelf is either preserved, dyed, or processed. Some of this stuff, even bugs won't eat. Why do we? Not even in the produce section are we safe; the fruits and vegetables have been grown in deficient soil and sprayed with pesticides. When the produce is picked, it is often dyed or waxed; and then, to add insult to injury, the grocer puts it under special lights to make it look fresh and wonderful.

Fat, Sugar, and Junk Food

As if this isn't bad enough, most Americans eat far too much fat, sugar, and junk food. Look into your neighbor's grocery cart when you are standing in the checkout line. For that matter, look into your own. What do you see? Candy, soda pop, baked goods, chips, dips, TV dinners, and the like. Americans are living off the "fat of the land"; and, as a result, they are suffering and dying from high blood pressure, heart disease, cancer, diabetes, and joint problems.

Lack of Exercise

What about exercise—are we burning any of these fat calories? Most of us sit all day in an office, ride in a car everywhere we go, and come home to eat and sit in front of the TV all evening. At least thirty minutes of exercise most days of the week is recommended by health professionals.

Alcohol and Drug Abuse

Then, there is all the alcohol abuse that is destroying lives. Alcohol can lead to impaired mental functions and destroy the liver, the kidneys, and the heart. In short, it can destroy the body. Liquor destroys on the highway, and it destroys in the home. How tragic that so many people think they cannot have a good time or "fit in" with the socially elite without liquor. This liquid drug has captured thousands in the clutches of addiction. I could also mention the devastation that other drugs are causing in our society.

Sexual Promiscuity

If what we Americans eat and drink isn't bad enough, what we do is just as bad. The "sexual revolution" and its legacies have brought sexually transmitted diseases that are running rampant across our nation. I don't know of any revolution that hasn't claimed lives, do you? The new morality is simply old sin, and *"the wages of sin is death"* (Romans 6:23 NKJV).

Stress

Those of us not sexually promiscuous are not guiltless when it comes to damaging our bodies. We put ourselves under immense stress "keeping up with the Joneses," making our fortunes, pursuing careers, worrying, and doing whatever else we do to put stress on ourselves. This leads to the next point, which is nonstop work.

Workaholism

We are a society of workaholics; it's work, work, work, work. While many people "burn the candle at both ends," they are burning up their bodies, as well.

In contrast, consider the second generation of Israelites who entered the Promised Land. They were born in the wilderness and couldn't push a cart around a supermarket. Their diet was manna for breakfast, manna for lunch, and manna for dinner. God provided them with very healthy food, and He provided refreshing water that gushed from the rock. Those Israelites also got plenty of exercise. They *walked* everywhere they went; for forty years they walked—from Egypt to the outskirts of Canaan and then all around the desert. When they finally entered the land of promise, they were "lean and mean," well able for the job ahead of them. Eating right, drinking plenty of water, getting enough rest, and exercising regularly make any people "lean and mean." However, when you walk down the streets of America today, you don't see the "lean and mean"; you see the fat and lazy.

The above are some of the major things we Americans are doing that hurt and damage us physically. We all want to be well, but we also want to do our own thing. People who are sick come for healing prayer, and they receive their miracles. Then, many of them go right out and continue to eat improperly, abuse alcohol, or mistreat their bodies in some other way and expect to keep their healings. It simply won't work that way. Everyone, without exception, will reap the consequences of his or her lifestyle. When the rules of good health are broken, the Lord is under no obligation to restore or maintain health in the one who abuses the body.

Although it is always God's pleasure to heal people, we see instances in the Bible when God did not heal. Let's review these occasions and determine why healing was withheld so that we can better understand the principles of healing and health for our own lives.

[There was] the case of King Jeroboam's sick son. Jeroboam knew he was in trouble with the Lord, but he still hoped that the prophet Ahijah would have a good word from God. However, this was not the case, and the boy died. (See 1 Kings 14:1–13.) There was at least one reason why the Lord withheld His healing hand....He saw something good in the child. God did not want this youngster to grow up in an evil, idolatrous environment and become like his father. God's love spared the child from such a fate. Don't forget that the Lord took the boy to a far *better* eternal existence. What was the cost of the king's sin? It was the life of one of his sons, the loss of the throne for his descendants, and essentially the end of the northern tribes of Israel as a kingdom. (See 1 King 14:14–16.)

[There was also] the death of King David's son, who was born of David's adulterous relationship with Bathsheba. This man cheated and murdered because of his fleshly appetites, but it cost him the life of the little prince. You see, not even kings can break God's rules without paying the consequences. Sin is sin wherever it is found, and it opens the door to satanic attack. Yet David didn't get bitter with God; instead, he got better. He found comfort in the knowledge that he would see his innocent son again in paradise, in spite of his sin. (See 2 Samuel 12:23.) Because of David's deep repentance, another son born of Bathsheba became king after him. Solomon was that son, and he ruled Israel at the pinnacle of its history.

Last, we look at the case of Gehazi, the servant of Elisha. This man served his master well until he was tempted by Naaman's riches. After Naaman was healed of leprosy, he wanted to reward Elisha with money and costly apparel. Elisha refused the Syrian general's gift because it was God who had healed him. Gehazi, however, just couldn't let this opportunity get away. He followed Naaman, thinking that Elisha would never know. Gehazi lied to Naaman, telling him that Elisha had changed his mind about the gift, and Naaman gave Gehazi some of the silver and clothing. To Gehazi's dismay, God showed the prophet what his servant had done. What did Gehazi pay for his stolen riches? He paid with his health. The leprosy of Naaman came upon his own body, and the Scriptures don't say that Gehazi repented or that he was ever healed. (See 2 Kings 5:20–27.)

A Recipe for Good Health

The above are sobering facts. Every action has a corresponding reaction. We cannot sin and abuse our bodies without experiencing the consequences.

Just because we feel well and seem to be in good health now doesn't mean we are going to stay that way. If we indulge our appetites, we will pay the price; and it won't be just at the cash register. Before you throw up your hands in despair, I want to give you a recipe you can follow to ensure good health. It isn't impossible—if you commit yourself to God and a good lifestyle.

The cause of eating right is not hopeless, nor is it cost prohibitive. You will spend more on junk food than you will on nutritious foods. Start reading labels, and eat lots of whole grains, fresh fruits, and vegetables. You can buy produce that is organically grown. Prepare meals from scratch and eliminate as much fat, sugar, and salt from your diet as possible. Reach for the water glass instead of the pop can or the beer can; water is the healthiest, most cleansing liquid you can drink.

Don't groan when I mention exercise. Remember, the Bible says that bodily exercise is profitable. (See 1 Timothy 4:8.) Now, it does say that exercise profits for only a little while, but your doctor will tell you the same thing. People can't expect to stay fit if they exercise only once in a while. I don't think any of us eats just one meal a week or sleeps only one night a week. Exercise is a necessity for good health. Any fitness program should include a reasonable amount of exercise. You don't need expensive equipment; walking is one of the very best exercises there is, and most of us have two legs. In years past, people got all the exercise they needed with physical labor, and they walked nearly every place they went.

What about rest? I don't believe it is impossible for the average American to get a sufficient amount of rest. God knows rest is necessary to maintain a healthy body. In every week, the Lord provided one day of rest for His people. Exodus 23:12 (NKJV) says, *"Six days you shall do your work, and on the seventh day you shall rest, that your ox and your donkey may rest, and the son of your female servant and the stranger may be refreshed."*

In spite of a very busy schedule, I find time to rest. Almost without exception, I am able to nap on a daily basis. If I work later than usual at the office, I have a little hideaway where I can lie down on the divan and nap. When I am flying to a Bible Encounter, I nap on the plane. During each Encounter, I find time every day to nap. If I'm overseas, I don't forget my nap. I've napped in airports and on planes, trains, and helicopters. I can nap anyplace, even on the floor. Do you think I'm a baby? Well, I've learned that in order to keep the pace I do and stay refreshed and alert to minister to people, I must include rest in my schedule. I don't believe your body is any different from mine.

If you consistently experience sleepless nights, the devil is robbing you of something that God guarantees. (See Proverbs 3:21–24.) Sleepless nights can be the result of eating the wrong thing or eating too close to bedtime, or of a fearful, angry, or fretful attitude. Memorize Scriptures, meditate on the Word, and pray during those sleepless periods, and cast all of your care on God. When you meditate on God's Word, the Word will lead you, keep you, and speak to you during your waking and sleeping moments. (See Proverbs 6:22.)

Next, how do we cope with stress? Stress is an awful thing. And although we may eliminate some things from our schedules, we all have some stress in our lives. Just normal daily routine puts some stress on our bodies and on our minds. If you are a workaholic, examine the things that are driving you to overwork. You must choose those activities in your schedule that have real, meaningful value and eliminate those things that don't. You don't need to be busy all the time to find self-worth. What will you have in the end if you kill yourself with work?

God has an answer for stress, too. Daily Bible reading and prayer will put your life into the proper perspective and help relieve stress. There is nothing like time spent with the Lord to put your mind and body at ease. Remember that you have a God who loves you enough to order your days. If you are a Spirit-filled Christian, you have the indwelling Holy Spirit who empowers you. He is also with you to guide and comfort you. Learn to rely on Him. The Lord has also given you approximately seven thousand Bible promises to help you through your day. Don't stress yourself with worry and fear; trust God. There is no better recipe for coping with stress.

Now, let's deal with the matter of sex. Many Americans think they are practicing "safe" sex, but the only safe sex is celibacy before marriage and fidelity in marriage. Any other sex is simply illicit, and the person who practices this type of lifestyle is bascially playing Russian roulette. The titillating little office affair, or any other affair, will cost the partners more than they bargained for. I am so grieved that our teenagers are being taught that it's okay if it's "safe." Today, the gay community is anything but gay. Homosexuals are dying from AIDS and many are infected with HIV, and yet many refuse to admit their perversion is sin. God loves these people, but they have opened their bodies to those things that God warns about. (See, for example, Romans 1:20–27.)

Some people who believe in God's miraculous, supernatural power to heal the sick have the notion that it is wrong to go to a doctor. I don't see that idea anywhere in the Bible. In Matthew 9:12 (NKJV), Jesus said, "*Those who are well have no need of a physician, but those who are sick.*" In other words, if you are sick, you may need a doctor. The beloved physician Luke was often a companion of Paul's, but I don't find anywhere that Paul rebuked him because of his earlier occupation. There is nothing evil about having periodic checkups or seeing a physician when you are ill. Will seeing the doctor or taking the medication he or she prescribes keep you from being healed if you are trusting God? Go to the doctor and get a diagnosis of your illness, and also see to it that you get prayer for healing. Then, you can go back to your doctor with a healthy body and testify to him of God's healing power.

Authority Power and Miracle-Working Power

To conclude, let's look at the nature of God's power to heal. If you were to read the New Testament in Greek, you would find two major words used to describe God's power. One of these words is *exousia*, and it means "authority" power. The other word is *dunamis*…and it means "miracle-working" power; *dunamis* is "dynamite" power.

God's Word is the *exousia*, or authority, of God, and it has great power. When a person believes and appropriates the Word, it can move and change circumstances because the Word is backed by the authority of almighty God. The One who framed the universe is the most powerful authority that exists. Every Christian has the authority of God's Word to believe for healing. Without that authority, we would have no right to expect healing.

Let me illustrate authority power. I know you have a healthy respect for that car with the revolving red and blue lights on top. Why is that? It is because the police officer behind the wheel has the authority to pull you over and make life uncomfortable if you have broken some traffic law. The officer wearing the badge doesn't have to physically drag you to traffic court. All he or she needs to do is write a ticket, and you will either have to pay the fine by mail or make a court appearance to contest the charge—at which point you will still have to pay the fine if the judge rules against you. The officer's vehicle and the badge the officer wears are symbols of the law that enforces his or her authority. God's Word is the highest law in the universe, and it is upheld by His authority power.

Now let's look at *dunamis* power. We are all familiar with what a few sticks of dynamite can do to the side of a mountain. The dynamite's explosive power will tear away tons of rock and soil. When the first atomic bomb was dropped, the entire world saw the destructive force of splitting the atom. Since then, that awesome power has held many people in nations all over the world in the grip of fear. However, it was God who created the atom. Did you know that Hebrews 1:2–3 says Jesus created the universe, and it is Jesus who holds all things *together* by the Word of His *dunamis* power? (See also Colossians 1:17.) The Lord has "dynamite" power ready to be released in miraculous ways for the benefit of all humanity. That miracle power is more than able to save souls, transform lives, and heal physical bodies.

The greatest dimension of God's miracle-working power was unleashed at the moment when life conquered death and Jesus was raised from the dead. Jesus gives that same power to believers when they are baptized with the Holy Spirit. (See Acts 1:8.) Every time someone is born again, every time someone is healed, God's miracle-working power is demonstrated. However, miracle-working power operates only in conjunction with authority power. If we expect to experience miracles, then we must be in line with God's authority. That authority is His Word.

Jesus always exercised both *exousia* and *dunamis* power when He healed and delivered the sick and demonized. The people marveled at His ability and said, "*What a word this is! For with authority and power He commands the unclean spirits, and they come out*" (Luke 4:36 NKJV). A Spirit-filled, born-again believer has been given that same ability. We have both the authority of God's Word and the miracle-working power of the Holy Spirit. Don't let the devil "do you in." Overcome him with the Word and the Spirit.

In Luke 10:19 (NKJV), Jesus gave believers authority power to overcome the evil powers of Satan when He said, "*Behold, I give you the authority [exousia] to trample on serpents and scorpions, and over all the power [dunamis] of the enemy, and nothing shall by any means hurt you.*" Although Satan also has supernatural power, he cannot exercise that power over Christians who know how to use the Word of God against him. You are able to overcome Satan by the blood of the Lamb and by the word of your testimony about Jesus as Savior, Redeemer, Healer, and Deliverer. (See Revelation 12:11.) Put the Word of God in your heart and in your mouth, and Satan must bow to that authority.

I have a practical illustration of *exousia* and *dunamis*. When my children were small, we sometimes left them with a babysitter. With my word, I gave the sitter authority to care for the children while we were gone. However, if Mike or Sarah did not obey her, I had a stick. That stick was small, but it was mighty. It had amazing *"dunamis"* power to keep those two in line. They knew both Wally and I had the parental authority to use the dynamite of that little stick.

To the religious hypocrites of His day, Jesus said, *"You are mistaken, not knowing the Scriptures nor the power [dunamis] of God"* (Matthew 22:29 NKJV). Even today, believers do not understand the necessity for the Word and the Spirit to work in agreement. Christians who are baptized with the Holy Spirit are enthusiastic about the miracle power of God. They expect to see *dunamis* at work in their lives and in others' lives, but they are often unwilling to come under the authority of God's Word in matters such as eating correctly, resting, and so forth. Their pat answer is, "I'm walking in the Spirit." These people don't believe God's rules apply to them because they think the Spirit supersedes the Word. However, the Word and the Spirit always agree! (See 1 John 5:7.)

On the other side of the coin are the fundamentalists who stand firm on the authority of God's holy Word. They claim to believe the Bible from cover to cover; they even believe the cover. These people will fight to preserve every comma and period; but when you talk to them about healing, they say, "Healing and miracles are not for today." Again, they believe that Jesus authenticated His Person and His ministry with the miraculous, but that there is no necessity for miracles today. Therefore, they rob themselves and others of God's miracle power and frustrate the grace of God. (See Galatians 2:21.) I'm convinced that no Christian would willingly sidestep the grace that was purchased for us at Calvary.

When believers don't allow the authority of the Word and the power of the Spirit to work together, they are out of balance. I want you to think of a bird. Can that bird get off the ground without two wings? Obviously not; nor can the bird sustain flight without the balance and strength of both wings. You, as a Christian, will never soar into the things of God unless you are balanced with the authority of God's Word and the miraculous, supernatural power of the Holy Spirit. Only with this balance can any one of us transcend the natural elements of this world and be elevated into the supernatural life of God.

I want to tell you about a woman who knew both the authority and the power of God. She exercised her faith in both areas and flew beyond the barriers of Satan and sickness into the healing, keeping power of Jesus. This lady shared her testimony in a service. Sometime previously, she had had a tumor removed from her back, but evidence of the tumor had reappeared. During the service, this lady felt the power of the Holy Spirit all over her, and she knew the tumor was gone. Moments later, the Lord showed me that someone in the audience had been healed of a tumor on the back. When I called out this healing, the woman responded. When her husband examined her back, all signs of the tumor were gone—never to return. Praise the Lord!

Christians who are not experiencing healing, or those who lose their healing, may not be living a balanced life. Some may not be accepting the reality of miracles, while others may not be coming under the authority of God's Word. First Corinthians 3:16 declares that our bodies are temples of God. However, multitudes of Christians ignore the warning in verse 17 (NKJV): *"If anyone defiles the temple of God, God will destroy him. For the temple of God is holy, which temple you are."* We wouldn't think of going into our church sanctuaries and defiling them in some way, such as spilling food and drink in them. However, we continually abuse our bodies with improper food and drink, lack of rest and exercise, and other bad habits that destroy the body. *"Do not be wise in your own eyes; fear the LORD and depart from evil. It will be health to your flesh, and strength to your bones"* (Proverbs 3:7–8 NKJV).

We must obey God's Word and care for our bodies correctly if we are to experience healing and continue to walk in health. When you were born again, your body became God's temple, and it belongs to Him. When you abuse your body, you are hurting God and preventing Him from continually activating health in your body. Often, people excuse their bad habits by saying they just can't quit. Yes, they can. It simply takes submitting our wills to God's will as we cast all our cares upon Him. (See James 4:7; 1 Peter 5:7.) All things are possible to the one who believes. (See Mark 9:23.) Let's all be bell ringers for God!

Journey into Word & Spirit

1. What lifestyle changes, such as reducing stress or altering your diet, do you believe God is calling you to make?

2. If you are ill as a result of sexual promiscuity or any kind of addiction, know that Jesus walked the earth saying to people, "I forgive you," "I heal you," and "Go and sin no more." Ask God to reveal His healing promise to you in the form of a specific Scripture, and then declare that Scripture out loud. He forgives all your sins and heals all your diseases.

3. Play some worship music and spend some time in prayer. Imagine that Jesus is with you in person, and ask Him to speak directly to your heart.

Chapter excerpted from Marilyn Hickey, *Total Healing* (New Kensington, PA: Whitaker House, 1992, 2011), chapter 10, "God's Dinner Bell Is Ringing."

About the Author

As founder and president of Marilyn Hickey Ministries, Marilyn is being used by God to help cover the earth with the Word. Her Bible teaching ministry is an international outreach via television, satellite, books, CDs, DVDs, and healing meetings. Marilyn has established an international program of Bible and food distribution, and she is committed to overseas ministry, often bringing the gospel to people who have never heard it before. She and her late husband, Wallace Hickey, founded the Orchard Road Christian Center in Greenwood Village, Colorado. Visit http://www.marilynandsarah.org/ for more information.

ASCENDING THE HIGH PLACES

Jerame Nelson

10

ASCENDING THE HIGH PLACES

Jerame Nelson

T he reason why we see so many miracles and salvations happen through us is because we keep the testimony of Jesus always before us. We talk about God stories. We anticipate that our friendship with Jesus will release greater encounters. And out of our intimate relationship, we just simply respond, "Lord, what do You want to do?" Then we say exactly what He says. We do what exactly what He wants to do. When we move in that realm of intimacy and obedience, the power of God shows up on a consistent basis.

⌒

Miranda and I were ministering at a church called Great Faith in Seoul, Korea; 3,000 to 4,000 hungry Koreans showed up every morning and every night, and God was also showing up to meet them in powerful ways. The first day of the meetings, ten deaf ears in a row opened up to total hearing. On the third or fourth day God prompted me to give a more specific altar call for people who had paralyzed right hands. I wondered how many people in the meeting could possibly fit that description, and to my surprise, seven people came forward. God healed five out of seven, on the spot, instantly. It seemed like we were ascending higher with God, drawing Heaven closer to earth as we ministered, experiencing creative miracles of a quantity and quality that we had not seen before. Something was different. And I asked the Lord what was going on.

During that trip, God visited me in a dream and gave me another key to unlock the future revolution of love.

In this dream, I was walking up this giant mountain, looking off into the distance as I hiked. The higher I got on the mountain, the clearer I could see in the valleys. Somehow I knew that it was the mountain of God.

After awhile, I looked toward the valley and saw a large tornado beginning to spin at a very high speed; everywhere it went it picked up trash and debris, and I could see it blowing around in the air. Yet it left something odd in its wake. Everywhere the tornado touched down, it left a golden brick road behind. It was so intriguing that I felt compelled to go higher so that I could see better. The adrenaline kicked in, and I practically ran up the mountain. To my surprise, a house sat near the top of the hill. So I went in the house and looked out the window. The storm was blowing closer, and I could see all the debris flying around, but I knew in my spirit it was a good storm. For some reason, I left the house and ran out the back door heading for the top of the hill. As often happens in dreams, right before I saw what happened next, I woke up.

Immediately upon waking, the Lord spoke to me and said, "Jerame, I want to send a powerful move of the Spirit to My people. I want to release a powerful move of the Spirit that will begin to affect entire regions. I want to release the winds of change in regions, in nations, and when I do this, it's going to take out all of the things that hinder the Church from the fullness of God—all the debris, all the trash, all that the enemy tries to toss in our way to hinder us. All the roadblocks are going to be removed, and there's going to be a clear path of the glory laid down for the people of God to walk on."

⌒

The mountain of God is an alone place. Like Jacob, you will have a secret place where you wrestle with angels and the supernatural. It's the place of encounter. It's a place of intimacy with God. Jesus would often leave His followers and the things of this world to ascend the mountain to pray. If He needed to be alone with His Father, how much more do we need to turn off the television and the video games and ascend the mountain to be with Him?

I'm reminded of the story when Jesus fed the five thousand. He took them on the mountain and gave thanks there. As He began to pass out bread, it multiplied. The miracle happened from the mountaintop. Jesus had a lifestyle of getting alone with His Father, and because of that, He always saw amazing words and miracles released through Him. Right after Jesus multiplied the bread, He sent His disciples to the other side of the Galilee and said He would meet them there.

He sent the disciples away, sent the people they fed away, and He went to the mountain by Himself with God. Instead of waiting until the disciples rowed halfway across the Sea of Galilee, He decided to walk to them on the water. He walked from the mountaintop onto the sea. Intimacy with God equals stepping into the supernatural. He walked up to the boat and freaked everybody out; they thought He was a ghost. But Peter said, "Lord, if it's really You, tell me to come." God wants us to ask Him things. God wants us to place a demand on the friendship we have with Him.

He wants us to say, "Lord, how do I do this? How do I walk? How do I live in the supernatural? How do I live in Your power?" Peter discovered a principle that God wants to give us. Do you want to know why he was able to walk on the water? Because he asked. And because God spoke it to him first, and said come.

Intimacy with God and obedience to His voice causes the manifestation of the supernatural. If you'll begin to live a lifestyle of ascending the hill of the Lord, a lifestyle of praying and intimacy with God, it will change who you are, and you will begin to walk in the supernatural.

⌣

Jesus walked around in great authority, healing and delivering people. In fact, He had more authority than any other person in His time, and the

Bible says that He would cast demons out with a word. Why could He do that when no one else could? Because He was being filled up on the top of the mountain with His God, and He was having encounters with the Holy Spirit where He began to shine in the glory. He carried the authority of Heaven that He obtained on the mountaintop back down into the earth and manifested it. We can, too. In fact, He is releasing His authority to you and to me to do even greater works than the ones Jesus did in the Bible. You need to spend time with Him—and then step out in faith.

One time I was in Hudson's Hope, British Columbia, where I was scheduled to be part of three days of revival meetings. During the first night of the meetings, I had a night off from speaking but went to support the other speakers and listen to what they had to share. The worship was awesome, and there was such a sweet presence of God in the room. I remember being so hungry for Jesus, all I wanted to do was worship Him. After the meeting ended, the conference hosts took me back to the home I was staying at and fed me, and I decided to turn in early as I was scheduled to preach first thing in the morning. Walking to my room, I thought about how good the worship was and how much I wanted to just be in the presence of God. I decided to put on my iPod and worship the Lord for a few minutes as I drifted off to sleep. So I close my eyes, listened to my iPod, and began to tell God how hungry I was to know Him more. After about two minutes of just softly praising the Lord, I felt the sweetest presence of God come into my room. Then it intensified. I opened my eyes, and much to my surprise, in the natural I could see what seemed to be a real glory cloud in my room.

It surrounded my bed, and I could feel God so strongly; it was like I was buzzing in the glory. This experience lasted for about five minutes, and then it faded away. This was the first time I had ever seen a glory cloud. In a state of great peace, I fell asleep and woke up the next day to get ready for the meetings.

That morning as I began to minister the Lord showed up in great power. A man who had hurt his back lifting a snowmobile was instantly healed as we prayed for him; another with arthritis was healed; and deafness left people's ears. Then bizarre miracles began to happen without anyone laying hands upon individuals. One little girl came up to me and asked, "Can God heal me too? I need my teeth to be healed." She smiled and showed me her really crooked teeth. Then I just said to her, "In the name of Jesus, be healed." I just spoke the word. I didn't even lay hands on her. She left, and I continued praying for others. A few minutes later she came up to me to show me that her teeth had been completely straightened out. It was awesome!

During the night session as I was preaching, the Lord told me that He was going to begin to sovereignly deliver people in His glory. He told me to stop preaching and release His presence. So I did exactly what He said.

I stopped preaching and prayed that God would release His glory into the room. When I did this, a woman on the left side of the platform fell on the ground and began screaming at the top of her lungs. Immediately the pastors ran over to her to see what was wrong with her and take control over the situation. As they did this, the Lord told me to tell them to stop and let the Lord have His way with her. So I told them what God has just said to me about her while the women kept screaming for a few more minutes. Suddenly, this amazing peace descended on her, and she was totally calm. I asked her what had happened. She then began to tell me that her whole life she had been attacked by demonic spirits of fear and anxiety. She had been to many deliverance specialists and had many powerful ministers pray for her, and no one could help her. Then, as we prayed and asked God to release His glory, she fell into a trance-like experience, and the Lord gave her revelation as to why she was always attacked and could not stop it.

In the vision she saw her grandmother hold her up to the sky and dedicate her life to satan. When her grandmother did this, she saw chains begin to bind her. As the vision continued, Jesus appeared with a sword and cut the chains off of her! She was instantly set free after this experience in the natural. Later, she testified to the people that she was fully set free from the fear and anxiety, and the attacks of the enemy for the first time in her whole life. You see, it was just like the passage we talked about earlier where Jesus' disciples could not cast a devil out of the little boy, but Jesus could because He had just been on the mountain with His Father.

I had just had my own encounter with God's glory cloud, and the results of that encounter were that miracle, signs, and wonders happened, and even this woman was set free from the demonic. We need to begin to ascend the mountain of God until we came into contact with the manifest presence of God. Then, when we come down off the mountain or out of our prayer time with God, we begin to carry the substance of the authority of Heaven into the natural realm of this earth and set others free from demonic strongholds, sickness, and disease. Authority is released when you encounter the glory of God.

⌣

Not Orphans

God wants us to understand that all things are possible with Him. He wants to change the way we think regarding our relationship with Him. Too many people think they have to *do* something to *get* something from God. God wants to crush the mentality of striving and release a greater revelation of His grace and love. We don't have to earn anything from God because Jesus went to the cross and declared, "It is finished." God has already given us everything regarding His kingdom. Ephesians 2:6 says that we are seated together in heavenly place with Jesus. God brought a new covenant to us, a covenant of the love of God. A lot of us haven't even wrapped our minds around the fact that we have a good Father in Heaven who longs to give good gifts to His children.

We are not orphans who have to beg for our needs. We don't have to try or strive to get things.

One woman who works with orphans has much to teach us about the orphan spirit. I remember listening to Heidi Baker talk about the kids at her orphanage in Mozambique. When children initially arrive at the Children's Center, poor, hungry, and unused to eating on a regular basis, they see the food set out on the table and go crazy. They jump on it and devour it. Even a month later, they are still jumping on it as if it will be their last meal. At first, Heidi asked the Lord what was going on with the children, and the Lord explained that they were not yet sons and daughters. The Lord said that they didn't understand that food was going to be there day after day because they never ate on a regular basis. They devoured everything they could quickly out of fear—because they didn't know when they would have their next meal.

That is the spirit of an orphan. By the time Heidi has had them for a couple of months, they know they are sons and daughters and that a meal is going to come every day. As they begin to come into a revelation of the Father's love through Rolland and Heidi Baker's ministry, they know that someone, Papa and Mama, is going to care for them.

We are much like the orphans of Mozambique. Many try to gobble up all they can—just for themselves. God wants us to stop acting like orphans running from conference to conference trying to devour everything we can. He wants to meet with you at your kitchen table, in your car, in your bedroom. He wants to meet with you wherever you will let Him meet with you. God especially wants to meet with you on the backside of the desert where you feel all alone.

Journey into Word & Spirit

1. The Father wants you to receive His love in the form of healing. But if you don't feel like a favored child, how can you receive it? If you feel like an "orphan," spend some time with the Lord and ask Him to minister to your estranged heart.

2. Put on some instrumental worship music and spend some time in prayer. Imagine that you are sitting next to Jesus on a mountaintop, when a cloud of glory moves over you and Jesus begins to speak to you about your healing. What is He saying to you?

Chapter excerpted from Jerame Nelson, *Manifesting God's Love through Signs, Wonders, and Miracles: Discovering the Keys of the Kingdom* (Shippensburg, PA: Destiny Image Publishers, Inc., 2010), 74, 77–78, 86–87, 98–101, 120–121.

About the Author

Jerame Nelson is a modern-day healing revivalist and popular conference speaker, and is based in Pasadena, California. Jerame and his wife, Miranda, founded Living at His Feet Ministries, which is dedicated to releasing the presence and power of God to heal and equip the saints around the world.

Jerame is the author of *Burning Ones* and several other books geared toward the 20- to 30-year-old emerging church. Visit www.livingathisfeet.org for more information.

FAITH FOR WHOLENESS

Smith Wigglesworth

11

FAITH FOR WHOLENESS

Smith Wigglesworth

I believe the Word of God is so powerful that it can transform any and every life. There is power in God's Word to make that which does not exist to appear. There is executive power in the words that proceed from His lips. The psalmist told us, "*He sent His word and healed them*" (Psalm 107:20 NKJV). Do you think the Word has diminished in its power? I tell you, it has not. God's Word can bring things to pass today as it did in the past.

The psalmist said, "*Before I was afflicted I went astray, but now I keep Your word*" (Psalm 119:67 NKJV). And again, "*It is good for me that I have been afflicted, that I may learn Your statutes*" (Psalm 119:71 NKJV). If our afflictions will bring us to the place where we see that we cannot "*live by bread alone, but by every word that proceeds from the mouth of God*" (Matthew 4:4 NKJV), they will have served a blessed purpose. I want you to realize that there is a life of purity, a life made clean through the Word He has spoken, in which, through faith, you can glorify God with a body that is free from sickness, as well as with a spirit set free from the bondage of Satan.

Around the pool of Bethesda lay a great multitude of sick folk—blind, lame, paralyzed—waiting for the moving of the water. (See John 5:2–4.) Did Jesus heal all of them? No, He left many around that pool unhealed. Undoubtedly, many had their eyes on the pool and had no eyes for Jesus. There are many today who always have their confidence in things they can see. If they would only get their eyes on God instead of on natural things, how quickly they would be helped.

The Bread of Healing

The following question arises: Is salvation and healing for all? It is for all who will press right in and claim their portion. Do you remember the case of that Syro-Phoenician woman who wanted the demon cast out of her daughter? Jesus said to her, *"Let the children be filled first, for it is not good to take the children's bread and throw it to the little dogs"* (Mark 7:27 NKJV). Note that healing and deliverance are here spoken of by the Master as *"the children's bread"* (NKJV); therefore, if you are a child of God, you can surely press in for your portion.

The Syro-Phoenician woman purposed to get from the Lord what she was after, and she said, *"Yes, Lord, yet even the little dogs under the table eat from the children's crumbs"* (Mark 7:28 NKJV). Jesus was stirred as He saw the faith of this woman, and He told her, *"For this saying go your way; the demon has gone out of your daughter"* (Mark 7:29 NKJV).

Today many children of God are refusing their blood-purchased portion of health in Christ and throwing it away. Meanwhile, sinners are pressing through and picking it up from under the table and are finding the cure, not only for their bodies, but also for their spirits and souls. The Syro-Phoenician woman went home and found that the demon had indeed gone out of her daughter. Today there is bread—there is life and health—for every child of God through His powerful Word.

The Word can drive every disease away from your body. Healing is your portion in Christ, who Himself is our bread, our life, our health, our All in All. Though you may be deep in sin, you can come to Him in repentance, and He will forgive and cleanse and heal you. His words are spirit and life to those who will receive them. (See John 6:63.) There is a promise in the last verse of Joel that says, *"I will cleanse their blood that I have not cleansed"* (Joel 3:21). This as much as says that He will provide new life within. The life of Jesus Christ, God's Son, can so purify people's hearts and minds that they become entirely transformed—spirit, soul, and body.

The sick folk were around the pool of Bethesda, and one particular man had been there a long time. His infirmity was of thirty-eight years' standing. Now and again an opportunity to be healed would come as the angel stirred the waters, but he would be sick at heart as he saw another step in and be healed before him. Then one day Jesus was passing that way, and seeing him lying there in that sad condition, He asked, *"Do you want to be made well?"* (John 5:6 NKJV). Jesus said it, and His words are from everlasting to everlasting. These are His words today to you, tried and tested one. You may say, like this poor sick man, "I have missed every opportunity up until now." Never mind that. *"Do you want to be made well?"*

Is It the Lord's Will?

I visited a woman who had been suffering for many years. She was all twisted up with rheumatism and had been in bed two years. I asked her, "What makes you lie here?" She said, "I've come to the conclusion that I have a thorn in the flesh." I said, "To what wonderful degree of righteousness have you attained that you must have a thorn in the flesh? Have you had such an abundance of divine revelations that there is a danger of your being exalted above measure?" (See 2 Corinthians 12:7–9.) She said, "I believe it is the Lord who is causing me to suffer." I said, "You believe it is the Lord's will for you to suffer, but you are trying to get out of it as quickly as you can. You have medicine bottles all over the place. Get out of your hiding place, and confess that you are a sinner. If you'll get rid of your self-righteousness, God will do something for you. Drop the idea that you are so holy that God has to afflict you. Sin is the cause of your sickness, not righteousness. Disease is not caused by righteousness, but by sin."

There is healing through the blood of Christ and deliverance for every captive. God never intended His children to live in misery because of some affliction that comes directly from the Devil. A perfect atonement was made at Calvary. I believe that Jesus bore my sins, and I am free from them all. I am justified from all things if I dare to believe. (See Acts 13:39.) *"He Himself took our infirmities and bore our sicknesses"* (Matthew 8:17 NKJV), and if I dare to believe, I can be healed.

See this helpless man at the pool. Jesus asked him, *"Do you want to be made well?"* (John 5:6 NKJV). But there was a difficulty in the way. The man had one eye on the pool and one eye on Jesus. If you will look only to Christ and put both of your eyes on Him, you can be made every bit whole—spirit, soul, and body. It is the promise of the living God that those who believe are justified, made free, from all things. (See Acts 13:39.) And *"if the Son makes you free, you shall be free indeed"* (John 8:36 NKJV).

You say, "Oh, if I could only believe!" Jesus understands. He knew that the helpless man had been in that condition for a long time. He is full of compassion. He knows about that kidney trouble; He knows about those corns; He knows about that neuralgia. There is nothing He does not know. He wants only a chance to show Himself merciful and gracious to you, but He wants to encourage you to believe Him. If you can only believe, you can be saved and healed. Dare to believe that Jesus was wounded for your transgressions, was bruised for your iniquities, was chastised that you might have peace, and that by His stripes there is healing for you here and now. (See Isaiah 53:5.) You have failed because you have not believed Him. Cry out to Him even now, *"Lord, I believe; help my unbelief!"* (Mark 9:24 NKJV).

I was in Long Beach, California, one day. I was with a friend, and we were passing by a hotel. He told me of a doctor there who had a diseased leg. He had been suffering from it for six years and could not get around. We went up to his room and found four doctors there. I said, "Well, doctor, I see you have plenty going on. I'll come again another day." I was passing by another time, and the Spirit said, "Go see him." Poor doctor! He surely was in poor shape. He said, "I have been like this for six years, and nobody can help me." I said, "You need almighty God." People are trying to patch up their lives, but they cannot do anything without God. I talked to him for a while about the Lord and then prayed for him. I cried, "Come out of him in the name of Jesus." The doctor cried, "It's all gone!"

Oh, if we only knew Jesus! One touch of His might meets the need of every crooked thing. The trouble is getting people to believe Him. The simplicity of this salvation is so wonderful. One touch of living faith in Him is all that is required for wholeness to be your portion.

I was in Long Beach about six weeks later, and the sick were coming for prayer. Among those filling up the aisle was the doctor. I said, "What is the trouble?" He said, "Diabetes, but it will be all right tonight. I know it will be all right." There is no such thing as the Lord's not meeting your need. There are no *ifs* or *mays*; His promises are all *shall*s. *"All things are possible to him who believes"* (Mark 9:23 NKJV). Oh, the name of Jesus! There is power in that name to meet every human need.

At that meeting there was an old man helping his son to the altar. He said, "He has fits—many every day." Then there was a woman with cancer. Oh, what sin has done! We read that when God brought forth His people from Egypt, *"there was not one feeble person among their tribes"* (Psalm 105:37). No disease! All healed by the power of God! I believe that God wants a people like that today.

I prayed for the woman who had the cancer, and she said, "I know I'm free and that God has delivered me." Then they brought the boy with the fits, and I commanded the evil spirits to leave in the name of Jesus. Then I prayed for the doctor. At the next night's meeting the house was full. I called out, "Now, doctor, what about the diabetes?" He said, "It is gone." Then I said to the old man, "What about your son?" He said, "He hasn't had any fits since." We have a God who answers prayer.

Sin and Sickness

Jesus meant this man at the pool to be a testimony forever. When he had both eyes on Jesus, He said to him, "Do the impossible thing. *'Rise, take up your bed and walk'* (John 5:8 NKJV)." Jesus once called on a man with a withered hand to do the impossible—to stretch forth his hand. The man did the impossible thing. He stretched out his hand, and it was made completely whole. (See Matthew 12:10–13.)

In the same way, this helpless man began to rise, and he found the power of God moving within him. He wrapped up his bed and began to walk off. It was the Sabbath day, and there were some folks who, because they thought much more of a day than they did of the Lord, began to make a fuss. When the power of God is being manifested, a protest will always come from some hypocrites. Jesus knew all about what the man was going through and met him again. This time He said to him, *"See, you have been made well. Sin no more, lest a worse thing come upon you"* (John 5:14 NKJV).

There is a close relationship between sin and sickness. How many know that their sicknesses are a direct result of sin? I hope that no one will come to be prayed for who is living in sin. But if you will obey God and repent of your sin and stop it, God will meet you, and neither your sickness nor your sin will remain. *"The prayer of faith will save the sick, and the Lord will raise him up. And if he has committed sins, he will be forgiven"* (James 5:15 NKJV).

Faith is just the open door through which the Lord comes. Do not say, "I was saved by faith" or "I was healed by faith." Faith does not save and heal. God saves and heals through that open door. You believe, and the power of Christ comes. Salvation and healing are for the glory of God. I am here because God healed me when I was dying, and I have been around the world preaching this full redemption, doing all I can to bring glory to the wonderful name of the One who healed me.

"Sin no more, lest a worse thing come upon you" (John 5:14 NKJV). The Lord told us in one place about an evil spirit going out of a man. The house that the evil spirit left got all swept and put in order, but it received no new occupant. That evil spirit, with seven other spirits more wicked than himself, went back to that unoccupied house, and *"the last state of that man [was] worse than the first"* (Matthew 12:45 NKJV).

The Lord does not heal you to go to a baseball game or to a racetrack. He heals you for His glory so that from that moment your life will glorify Him. But this man remained stationary. He did not magnify God. He did not seek to be filled with the Spirit. And his last state became *"worse than the first."*

The Lord wants to so cleanse the motives and desires of our hearts that we will seek one thing only, and that is His glory. I went to a certain place one day and the Lord said, "This is for My glory." A young man had been sick for a long time. He had been confined to his bed in an utterly hopeless condition. He was fed with a spoon and was never dressed. The weather was damp, so I said to the people in the house, "I wish you would put the young man's clothes by the fire to air." At first they would not take any notice of my request, but because I was persistent, they at last got out his clothes. When they had been aired, I took them into his room.

The Lord said to me, "You will have nothing to do with this," and I just lay prostrate on the floor. The Lord showed me that He was going to shake the place with His glory. The very bed shook. I laid my hands on the young man in the name of Jesus, and the power fell in such a way that I fell with my face to the floor. In about a quarter of an hour, the young man got up and walked back and forth praising God. He dressed himself and then went out to the room where his father and mother were. He said, "God has healed me." Both the father and mother fell prostrate to the floor as the power of God surged through that room. There was a woman in that house who had been in an asylum for lunacy, and her condition was so bad that they were about to take her back. But the power of God healed her, too.

The power of God is just the same today as it was in the past. Men need to be taken back to the old paths, to the old-time faith, to believing God's Word and every "Thus says the Lord" in it. The Spirit of the Lord is moving in these days. God is coming forth. If you want to be in the rising tide, you must accept all God has said.

"*Do you want to be made well?*" (John 5:6 NKJV). It is Jesus who asks this question. Give Him your answer. He will hear, and He will answer.

Journey into Word & Spirit

1. Have you prayed "Lord, I believe; help my unbelief"? Accept healing as your portion in Christ, who is your health and your life, and press in to receive your portion.

2. Will you be made whole? Saying yes and declaring the scriptural promises of God for healing out loud will activate your faith.

3. Do you know that God has forgiven your sins, and that because of that, you can forgive others for the sins they have committed against you? Forgiveness breaks the chains of sickness. Spend some time with the Lord breaking those chains.

Chapter excerpted from Smith Wigglesworth, *Smith Wigglesworth on Healing* (New Kensington, PA: Whitaker House, 1999), chapter 23, "Do You Want to Be Made Well?"

About the Author

Smith Wigglesworth (1859–1947), known as the Apostle of Faith, had an international evangelistic and healing ministry. A plumber by trade, Wigglesworth had a dramatic life change when, at age forty-eight, he was baptized in the Holy Spirit and anointed with power for preaching and healing. Signs and wonders characterized his ministry. His unquenchable faith inspired thousands to receive salvation, healing, and the filling of the Holy Spirit.

THE THREE PARTIES
CONCERNED IN
YOUR HEALING

Aimee Semple McPherson

12

THE THREE PARTIES CONCERNED IN YOUR HEALING

Aimee Semple McPherson

There are three parties concerned in your divine healing—you, the Lord Jesus, and the one who prays for you. Let us consider just what part each must take in order to bring about your healing. The first to be concerned in your healing is, of course, you.

You

If you want to be cleansed and made completely whole, you have a part to do in pressing through the thronging doubt, hindrances, and materialism of the day and touching the hem of the Master's robe. So often, people come to me for prayer who have only a passive faith and are dumbly *hoping* that I can heal them or do all the interceding on their behalf. Though the hands of everyone about them may be lifted in intercession, their faces wet with tears, and a real prayer of faith in their hearts, such ones stand passively—without any real soul outcry to God, waiting for our prayers to heal them and *hoping* it will be done. If they are healed, they will be grateful to those who prayed and say that they *certainly had some kind of power.* If not healed, they will go out and criticize the meeting, telling the people that they *tried it* or *had a treatment* but that it did them no good.

But do you not see that people like this have not done their part in pressing through to Jesus with active faith and believing prayer? You can *try* doctors, *try* medicine, *try* science, *try* baths and electric treatment, but you cannot *try* Jesus Christ. Remember also that neither Christ nor His servants who pray for you give "treatments." That word belongs to doctors or to Christian Science but has no place in the Bible or in these revival meetings. The very fact that one uses this word in this connection would indicate that his heart is far from God and that the truth concerning the atonement and power of the slain Lamb of Calvary is not in him.

The one coming for healing has a real, definite part to play in his coming to the Great Physician.

The disciples had to come to land before they could be warmed at the fire that Jesus had kindled or partake of the fish He had broiled. They had to leave their ship, come to shore, and draw near to Jesus before they could receive the bounties from His hand. You, too, must come out of the ship in which you have gone "fishing" for worldly joys and gains, toiling through the night and catching nothing. Let down your nets on the right side; prove the bounty of His goodness, love, and power; and then jump overboard, like Peter, when his Master bade him, "Come and dine." (See John 21:3–12.)

The prodigal son had to come home before he could receive the kiss of reconciliation, the ring, the best robe, and the shoes for his weary wandering feet. The father could not carry the best robe to his son when he sat among the swine, eating the husks that they did eat. The father could not meet the son on the ground of his prodigality; the son had to return to his father's home and meet him on his own just and righteous ground. Besides, the best robe would soon have been soiled and besmirched, discrediting his father's name, had it been worn in the midst of his reveling and merrymaking. (See Luke 15:11–24.)

Just so, if you want to be made whole and receive the best robe and gifts the heavenly Father has to give—salvation, healing, and the baptism of the Holy Spirit, through the Lord Jesus Christ—you, too, must do your part, leave the land of sin and backsliding (your soul is sick of it all, anyway), and say, "I will arise and go." Come, crying, "Father, I have sinned against heaven and in Your sight." Through the mist of penitent tears, you will surely see the Father running to meet you with clothing, with food, and with gladness. Just as the ring that the father gave the son had no ending but was a complete circle, so the love, promises, and provision of Christ are unending, for He is the same today as He was yesterday and as He will be evermore.

Naaman had to dip seven times in the Jordan before he was cleansed of his leprosy. He had his part to play in obedience and humility. Had Naaman failed to do his part, God could not have done His, and he would have gone away uncleansed. Naaman did not go part of the way to the Jordan but all the way; he dipped not three or four but seven times. If he dipped the first two or three times with the thought of a *treatment* in his mind, the thought was surely washed away before he went down the seventh time in obedience and faith, for he came up every bit whole. (See 2 Kings 5:1–14.)

Many come for healing today just like Naaman went to Elisha. They think they can sit outside in their chariot or automobile and have God's servant run out and heal them. No, no! Rich or poor, bond or free, all must go the same humble road to the Jordan. It is not the servant but the Master who has the power.

The importance of the work of preparation cannot be spoken of too highly or be too greatly emphasized.

People who come blindly, rushing into the meetings, saying that they have heard "there is a miracle woman here who can heal them at once" and that they want to be *treated* at once so they can catch the next train for business and pleasure are quickly disillusioned. First of all, they are informed that there is no "miracle woman" here at all, only a simple little body whom the Lord has called from a milk-pail on a Canadian farm, bidding her to tell the good news of a Savior who lives and loves and answers prayers.

Then they are told to settle themselves down and take part in the meetings, just as though they were going to any great hospital for an operation and were preparing for it for days, obeying each order. So they are told to prepare their house before coming into the presence of Jesus, the Great Physician. They are reminded that if they rush into a hospital, dirty and dusty and travel-stained, demanding that a serious, major operation should be performed that instant, in order that they might catch the next train for home, the doctors would explain to them that they were in no condition to go to the table as they were, lest infection should set in and their latter condition be more serious than the former.

How clean and purged their systems must be before going to the operating table! Then, how clean and pure their hearts and lives must be before coming to ask the sacred and holy touch of Christ upon their mortal bodies.

How clean the nurse would bathe them—how sterile and white the robe she would dress them in before they were wheeled to the operating table! How pure, then, they must be, spiritually washed in the blood of Jesus and clad in the white robes of righteousness, beneath which heart and life and soul are made pleasing in His sight, before coming for healing.

The results of this preparation are self-evident. They are wonderful. Cancers have disappeared, fibroid tumors have melted like snow before the sun, goiters have gone down like a toy balloon that is punctured, stiff limbs have been made to bend, blind eyes have recovered sight, deaf ears have been unstopped, dumb lips have been opened, and withered arms have come to life and grown several inches in an hour.

Are you a real Christian—a follower of the Lamb? Have you been born again? Are you taking up your cross daily, denying yourself, and following after Him? Is your life counting for God and souls? Even when the wires of heavenly connection are up, you should inspect them carefully before coming for healing. It takes only a little bit of paper in the electric light socket to keep the light from shining. It takes only a little doubt, hardness, backbiting, criticism, unforgiveness, disobedience, or a grudge to hinder the blessed power of God from flowing into that life of yours. It is a very sacred thing to ask the divine touch of Jesus upon these mortal bodies of ours. There is no question as to the power being in the storehouse or as to our electric lightbulb needing the power; but, oh, make sure of the connection!

"Yes, yes," I hear someone cry, "I see that I have a real part to fill if I would receive my healing, but it has been so many years since I went to church or have taken any real interest in religion; just what must I do to be healed?"

Brother, Sister, dear, I trust that the first step you will take will be to fall so in love with Jesus the crucified that the healing of your body will be a secondary consideration. Seek first the kingdom of God and His righteousness, and all these things will be added unto you. (See Matthew 6:33.) Come to the altar, get down on your knees today, repent of your sins, turn to the Lord, and seek salvation.

"Oh, Sister, not at that altar!" someone exclaims. "Not here, where I am so well-known! People will talk about it so. I can pray better in my own room by my own bedside, I am quite sure."

Why, that is just what Naaman said: *"Are not Abana and Pharpar, rivers of Damascus, better than all the waters of Israel? may I not wash in them, and be clean?"* (2 Kings 5:12). Yet none other than those lowly, humble, despised waters brought healing to the leper. You have tried your own way and gotten but deeper into sorrow; why not come God's way—the way of the humble and lowly Nazarene who hung on the cross for you? Repent of your sins with a godly sorrow for sin. Do not glaze over the surface but go to the depths.

"Seek My face," calls the Savior. Oh, let your heart answer, "Your face, O Lord, will I seek." (See Psalm 27:8.) Hear the Master sweetly say, "Draw near unto Me, and I will draw near unto you." (See James 4:8.)

Why, He is running to meet you already with wide-open arms. "Poor, weary, sin-sick child," He is saying, "you have been wandering such a long, long time. You have been torn by the thorns and bruised by the jagged rocks. None other has been able to fill the hungry longing of your heart. Come closer to Me, child. Turn your back upon the world, with its bitterness and sin. Come closer to My wounded side and lay your head upon My breast. I will pardon your backsliding. I will forgive you freely. A clean heart will I give you, and a new spirit will I create within you. Your sins will I cast into the sea of My forgetfulness and remember them against you nevermore. Your cup will I fill to overflowing with the joy of salvation, and your head will I anoint with the oil of gladness. Seek My face, dear child! Let Me be your all and in all."

Glory to Jesus! When you get there, dear heart, the healing of your body will be but a secondary thought.

> Since mine eyes were fixed on Jesus,
> I've lost sight of all beside
> So enchained my spirit's vision,
> Gazing at the crucified.[1]

It is not money, nor arrogance, nor even hope that makes them clean and white, but implicit faith, humility, and obedience to the voice of the Lord.

The railroad track must be laid—every tie in place, every rail fastened, and the last spike driven, before the great transcontinental express can go through. It takes a great deal longer to lay the track than for the express to pass by.

In coming for healing, make sure of the condition of the track. You are inviting the express of God's unlimited power to come over. Remember that, in making railroads, the hills must be laid low and the valleys exalted; pride must flow down before Him, and the rough places must be made smooth. Do not spend so much time worrying and scolding because the train does not come more quickly. *You* care for the track—*God* will take care of the train.

Take the electric light, for instance. It is not enough to have an electric lightbulb in your possession—the wires must be strung and the connections properly made clear back to the powerhouse before the light can shine in your home.

Just so, it is not enough for you to say, "I have a body that needs healing, and I know that the Lord has the power to make me whole." That is like saying, "I have an electric lightbulb in my hand, and I know there is enough current in the powerhouse to make it a shining light, but what about the wires and connections between?"

Selfish motives are gone, and you are now drawing nearer every moment to the Great Physician who has power to heal the sick. The all-absorbing love for your newfound Christ and the overwhelming desire to be pleasing in His sight and to win jewels for His crown have taken the place of selfishness.

---

1. Mary D. James, "All for Jesus," 1871.

"And does this hinder one from seeking physical healing," you ask, "seeing that our eyes have been taken off our own suffering and fixed upon Christ?"

Ah, no! It will help you a thousand miles along the way. For, instead of asking healing for a selfish motive only, one now seeks life and strength, that one may the more fully and gladly serve and win other souls for this adorable Christ of Calvary.

The conflict is over, the battle ended. There is a *nevertheless not my will but Thine be done* in the soul. (See Luke 22:42.) "Dear Jesus, if You want me to go to heaven, I thank You that I know it is well with my soul. But if, oh Lord, it is Your will to spare me on this earth, I pray that I may have the strength and health, the power and wisdom, to win my family and others for You, dear Savior, and to be a shining light to those who sit in darkness."

If it is His good will to take one of the children home—amen! If not, bless the Lord, you can touch the hem of the Master's robe and have healing and strength for His service today, even as did they who lived when Jesus walked this earth. But whatsoever you do, whether you eat or drink, seek healing and strength, be sure that you do all for the glory of God. (See 1 Corinthians 10:31.) You can then look up as you come to the altar and, lifting your hands toward heaven, say:

> My body, soul and spirit
> Jesus, I give to Thee,
> A consecrated offering,
> Thine evermore to be.
> My all is on the altar,
> I'm waiting for the fire;
> Waiting, waiting, waiting,
> I'm waiting for the fire.[2]

Then remember, if you bring your gift to the altar and there remember that your brother has something against you, leave your gift before the altar and go first to be reconciled to your brother. Then come and offer your gift. (See Matthew 5:23–24.)

And when you stand praying, forgive—make those old-time grudges right. Go make it right with that one to whom you have not spoken for so

2. Mary D. James, "Consecration," 1869.

long. Ask your wife to forgive the harsh words that have so often made the tears spring into her eyes. Forgive that enemy the injury you could never forgive before. (See Mark 11:25.) Otherwise, how can you pray, "Forgive us our trespasses, as we forgive those who trespass against us"? (See Matthew 6:12.)

"But what has all this to do with my receiving healing?" you ask. "I thought that all I had to do was to walk right up on that platform, be prayed for, and be healed without further obligation on my part. What has all this to do with it, anyway?"

Why, don't you see, this is the stringing of the electric light wires between the bulb and the powerhouse and the making sure of the proper connections. This is the laying of the track across the desert wastes or the tunneling through the mountains and making straight paths for His feet so that the mighty express of God's glory and power may pass through.

Seek *first* the kingdom of God and His righteousness, and all else will be added unto you. Put first things first. Spend time in prayer. Read your Bible carefully and prayerfully, especially Matthew, Mark, Luke, John, and the Acts of the Apostles, with reference to those whom Jesus healed, and see what part they had in obeying His command and in having active faith.

Establish family worship in your home. Do not wait till you are here but begin to serve Jesus even now, till joy and peace are flooding your heart. Faith is rising mountain-high, and you have *prayed through* and gotten the witness; every wire is in place between the bulb and the powerhouse, and you are ready for the hand of prayer to turn the switch and let the current of God's power flow through.

Jesus

The next and greatest one concerned in your healing is, of course, the one to whom you are coming for healing—Jesus. Has He the power to heal? Is He willing to do so, and will He do His part?

Yes; beyond a doubt, He has the same power today as He had in the old days. His promises are constant. Amen to everyone who believes. When the leper in the Bible days said, *"If thou wilt, thou canst make me clean"* (Mark 1:40), and his healing depended upon the "willingness of Jesus," the Master, without hesitation, said, *"I will; be thou clean"* (Mark 1:41). There is no doubt as to His *willingness*, if we only have the faith and ask for His glory.

As for Jesus *doing His part*, Brother, Sister, it was already done when He purchased our healing at the cruel whipping post…, that, by His stripes, we might be healed (see 1 Peter 2:24), for *"himself took our infirmities, and bare our sicknesses"* (Matthew 8:17).

Just as in salvation, Christ has done *His* part in the finished work of Calvary and now awaits our coming to the cross in faith to accept and make this great redemption ours, so with divine healing, the Great Physician, the Son of Righteousness with healing in His wings, has done His part. He bore the cruel lash, carried our pain and suffering, was smitten of God and afflicted as our burden-bearer, and bore not only our sins but that dire result of sin—sickness and pain. Thus, with Isaiah, we can cry exultingly, *"He was wounded for our transgressions…and with his stripes we are healed"* (Isaiah 53:5).

Indeed, He will do His part. Draw near to Him, and He will draw near to you. (See James 4:8.) Reach out your hands in faith and touch the blessed hem of His garment, and He will bend low over you. You will feel the gentle pressure of His nail-pierced hand laid in healing and benediction upon your head. Jesus is the same yesterday, today, and forever; He who heard the cry of His people in times past is just the same today. His ear has not grown heavy, that He cannot hear, nor has His arm been shortened, that it cannot save. (See Isaiah 59:1.)

The One Who Prays for You

The third party concerned in your healing is the one who anoints you with oil, according to James 5:14, and prays with you, that you might be made whole. Just what part is played by this one who prays for the sick, and of what importance is his role?

The first duty of the one who is instrumental in praying for the sick is the duty that Christ laid upon His disciples in John 10:49—namely, that of bringing the man near to Him. The blind man cried, *"Thou son of David, have mercy on me"* (Mark 10:47). He had faith. He had prayed through and reached the ear of the Master.

He had done his part.

Jesus was ready to do His part.

But a blessed duty, or part, in the healing was granted to the disciples when Jesus commanded them to bring the man near to Him. First, then, lift up Jesus from the earth. Talk of His power; magnify His name. Many take so much time talking about what Jesus *cannot* do that they spend very little time telling of the things He *can* do.

Sow the seed of faith in the hearts of the people, and have faith *yourself.* Those who pray for the healing of the sick should themselves first be partakers of the fruit and be a living example of what they preach, having a sound, whole body, and being invigorated by the strength and resurrection of the life of Jesus.

Bring the sufferer near to Christ in prayer, faith, and praise. Make Jesus so real through the preached Word that your audience can see His blessed face through the parting clouds and reach out their hands to touch Him.

Second, it is the sacred duty of those who pray for the sick to believe with the whole heart and have the real touch of God upon them, the Holy Spirit dwelling within them, and the authority of the Master clothing them as the raiment of Elijah clothed Elisha.

Let him ask in faith, nothing wavering. For he that wavereth is like a wave of the sea driven with the wind and tossed. For let not that man think that he shall receive any thing of the Lord. A double minded man is unstable in all his ways. (James 1:6–8)

One can tell in a moment whether a preacher, or the one who is exhorting or praying, has faith. Have you ever heard a man preach a long sermon and then say, "Now, *if* there is one here tonight who wants salvation, will you lift your hand and say, 'Pray for me'?"

Why, right there, his faith has wavered; he seldom gets more than the one he asked for, whereas the man of faith has won the day and cries, "Let *every* sinner or backslider in this building lift up your hand high, and by that lifted hand, say, 'Pray for me; *I* am a sinner and want salvation.' You all need Jesus! Let everyone lift his hands and say so." Have you watched the hands go up? And have you seen the hundreds of penitents weeping their way to the altars? So it is in the prayer for the sick. According to your faith, so will it be done to you.

In a recent meeting, we came to the closing day, and thousands were still waiting to be prayed for, so it became necessary for various groups, composed of some twenty ministers, to be called upon to offer prayer for the healing of the afflicted. Among the long lines of sufferers came a deaf man, desiring prayer that his hearing might be restored. A certain dear minister, who perhaps had never before been called upon to pray for deaf ears to be unstopped, began to talk to the Lord about His power and willingness to hear the prayers of His people. After a few moments, he looked at the man and, realizing that something definite should be done, leaned over inquiringly, brought his lips close to the ear in question, and asked, "O deaf ear, are you going to open? Are you?" Right there, he had wavered, and let not that man who wavers think that he will obtain anything from God! With the unction and power of the Holy Spirit upon him, he should have commanded, "O deaf ear, in the name of the Lord Jesus Christ, I *command* you to be opened and to hear the Word of the Lord! You deaf spirit, come out of him, in the mighty name of Jesus." Ask in faith, nothing wavering, and it will be done *according to your faith.*

Tell the one for whom you pray to have faith also, reaching out and clasping the promise to hold it tightly, and it will be his. Whether he is healed instantly or gradually, he must believe from that very hour.

Third, the one who prays for the sick should have clean hands and a pure heart.

Many ministers we know are using tobacco. Throw it away; let your own heart be cleansed with the precious blood and your lips be sweet and pure before you pray reverently the prayer of faith. Could you imagine Jesus smoking a big cigar and then going in to pray for the afflicted?

Do not expect to spend your time telling or listening to foolish, idle stories or gossip, or being a good mixer in the club, and then rushing into His presence to bring the power down. Keep close to Jesus yourself. Keep the lamp of faith brightly burning. Walk with God like Enoch of old, till your life is swallowed up in His own blessed will. Let triumphant faith mount up and up till your own face is all aglow, and poor, weak, tempest-driven souls see in you that mighty, unwavering confidence and trust in God that will give new courage and guide them into the calm, safe harbor of the Savior's strength and blessing.

Do not feel, however, dear, afflicted soul, that unless the preacher or elder who prays does his part, that you need necessarily go away without healing. Many are healed in answer to their own prayers while seated in the audience or while praying in their homes. *"Is any among you afflicted? let him pray"* (James 5:13). Even though you are alone, you can reach up right where you are and claim the promise. It is only natural, however, and perfectly scriptural, to want someone to pray the prayer of faith for you and to hold up your hands in encouragement as you come to God, for we also read:

> *Is any sick among you? let him call for the elders of the church; and let them pray over him, anointing him with oil in the name of the Lord: and the prayer of faith shall save the sick, and the Lord shall raise him up, and if he have committed sins, they shall be forgiven him.* (James 5:14–15)

Let us, therefore, do our part. Press in close to the Master—the Great Physician—the Shepherd of the sheep, who stands waiting with his flask of oil to make us whole in body, soul, and spirit. There is not a tear so blinding, but Jesus can wipe it away. There is not a hurt so deep in the heart, but He can comfort and bless. There is not a body so weary, so weak, and so sick, but His touch can strengthen and heal. There is not a load so heavy or a burden so great, but His love can lift and bear it away.

Journey into Word & Spirit

1. Are any doubts or other sins keeping you from touching the hem of the Master's robe for healing so that the "connection" between you and Him will be strong and clear? If so, repent of them and ask the Lord to set you free from those bondages.

2. Christ finished His work on the cross at Calvary, bearing your pain and suffering. So don't lose hope! Ask the Lord that His will be done in your life, and then find rest in His arms of love.

3. Put first things first—seek first God's kingdom and righteousness, and develop a deep love for the Lord.

Chapter excerpted from Aimee Semple McPherson, *Divine Healing Sermons* (New Kensington, PA: Whitaker House, 2014), chapter 4, "The Three Parties Concerned in Your Healing."

About the Author

In 1915, Aimee Semple McPherson began traveling around the United States, holding tent revivals, with some crowds reaching well over thirty thousand people. As an evangelist who preached the gospel not only across the United States but also around the world, "Sister Aimee" incorporated the cutting-edge communications media of her day, becoming a pioneer in broadcasting the gospel on the radio.

Upon opening the doors of Angelus Temple in Los Angeles in 1923, Sister Aimee developed an extensive social ministry, feeding more than 1.5 million people during the Great Depression. She summarized her message into four major points, which she called "the Foursquare Gospel." She founded the International Church of the Foursquare Gospel, also known as The Foursquare Church, which continues to spread the Foursquare Gospel throughout the world to this day.

"BEHOLD, I GIVE YOU POWER"

John G. Lake

13

"BEHOLD, I GIVE YOU POWER"

John G. Lake

"When he was come down from the mountain, great multitudes followed him. And, behold, there came a leper and worshipped him, saying, Lord, if thou wilt, thou canst make me clean."
—Matthew 8:1–2

That man knew that Jesus had the power to heal him, but he did not know it was God's will and that Jesus had committed Himself to the healing of mankind. If he had known, he would have said, "Lord, heal me."

It is always God's will to heal. Our faith may fail. My faith failed to the extent that unless someone else had gone under my life and prayed for me, I would have died. But God was just as willing to heal me as He could be. It was my faith that broke down. God is willing, just as willing to heal as He is to save. *Healing is a part of salvation.* It is not separate from salvation. Healing was purchased by the blood of Jesus. This Book always connects salvation and healing. David said:

Bless the LORD, *O my soul, and forget not all his benefits: who forgiveth all thine iniquities; who healeth all thy diseases.*   (Psalm 103:2–3)

There never has been a man in the world who was converted and was sick at the same time, that might not have been healed if he had believed God for it. But he was not instructed in faith to believe God for healing.

Supposing two men came to the altar. One is sick and lame; the other is a sinner. Suppose they knelt at the altar together. The sinner says, "I want to find the Lord." All in the house will immediately lend the love of their hearts and the faith of their souls to help him touch God. But the lame fellow says, "I have a lame leg" or "My spine is injured; I want healing." Instead of everybody lending their love and faith in the same way to the man, everybody puts up a question mark.

That comes because of the fact that we are instructed on the Word of God concerning the salvation of the soul, but our education concerning sickness and His desire and willingness to heal had been neglected. We have gone to the eighth or the tenth grade or the university on the subject of salvation, but on the subject of healing, we are in the ABC class.

Jesus put forth his hand, and touched him, saying, I will; be thou clean.
     (Matthew 8:3)

Did he ever say anything in the world but "I will"? Did He ever say, "I cannot heal you because it is not the will of God" or "I cannot heal you because you are being purified by this sickness" or "I cannot heal you because you are glorifying God in this sickness"? There is no such instance in the Book.

On the other hand, we are told, "He healed *all* that came to Him." (See Matthew 4:24; 8:16; 12:15; Luke 4:40; 6:19.) Never a soul ever applied to God for salvation or healing that Jesus did not save and heal! Did you ever think of what calamity it might have been if a man had come to Jesus once and said, "Lord, save me," and the Lord had said, "No, I cannot save you"? Every man forevermore would have a question mark as to whether God would save him or not. There would not be universal confidence, as there is today.

Suppose Jesus had ever said to a sick man, "No, I cannot heal you." You would have the same doubt about healing. The world would have settled back and said, "Well, it may be God's will to heal that man or that woman, but I do not know whether it is His will to heal *me*."

Jesus Christ did not leave us in doubt about God's will, but when the church lost her faith in God, she began to teach people that maybe it was not God's will to heal them. So the church introduced the phrase "If it be Thy will" concerning healing. But Jesus healed all who came to Him. (See Matthew 4:23; Luke 9:6, 11.)

Notice what it says in Isaiah:

*He will come and **save** you. **Then** the eyes of the blind shall be opened, and the ears of the deaf shall be unstopped. **Then** shall the lame man leap as an hart, and the tongue of the dumb sing.* (Isaiah 35:4–6)

Salvation and healing connected!

That it might be fulfilled which was spoken by Esaias the prophet, saying, Himself took our infirmities, and bare our sicknesses. (Matthew 8:17)

And lest we might be unmindful of that great fact that *"he hath borne our griefs [sicknesses, infirmities], and carried our sorrows"* (Isaiah 53:4), Peter emphasized it by saying,

Who his own self bare our sins in his own body on the tree, that we, being dead to sins, should live unto righteousness: by whose stripes ye were healed. (1 Peter 2:24)

Not "by whose stripes ye *are* healed," but *"by whose stripes ye **were** healed."* The only thing that is necessary is to *believe* God. God's mind never needs to act for a man's *salvation*. He gave the Lord and Savior Jesus Christ to die for you. God cannot go any farther in expressing His will in His desire to save man. The only thing that is necessary is to believe God. There is salvation by blood. There is salvation by power that actually comes from God into a man's life. The blood provided the power. Without the blood there would have been no power. Without the sacrifice there never would have been any glory. Salvation by blood, salvation by power.

The church in general is very clear in her faith on the subject of salvation through the sacrifice of the Lord and Savior Jesus Christ. Christians in general, regardless of their personal state of salvation, have a general faith and belief in the Lord and Savior Jesus Christ for the salvation of the world. But they are ever in doubt and very inexperienced on the power of God.

> *When he was come down from the mountain, great multitudes followed him. And, behold, there came a leper and worshipped him, saying, Lord, if thou wilt, thou canst make me clean. And Jesus put forth his hand, and touched him, saying, I will; be thou clean. And immediately his leprosy was cleansed. And Jesus saith unto him, See thou tell no man; but go thy way, show thyself to the priest, and offer the gift that Moses commanded, for a testimony unto them.* (Matthew 8:1–4)

Did you ever stop to think that there is no medical remedy for the real things that kill folks? Typhoid fever: Fill the patient with a tank full of medicine, and he will go right on for twenty-one days.

In 1913, I was in Chicago in a big meeting, when I received a telegram from the hospital in Detroit, saying, "Your son, Otto, is sick with typhoid fever. If you want to see him, come." I rushed for a train, and when I arrived, I found him in a ward. I told the man in charge I would like a private ward for him, so I could get a chance to pray for him. Well, God smote that thing in five minutes. I stayed with him for a couple of days until he was up and walking around. He went along for four or five weeks, and one day, to my surprise, I got another telegram telling me he had a relapse of typhoid.

So I went back again. This time there was no sunburst of God like the first time. Everything was as cold as steel, and my, I was so conscious of the power of the devil that I could not pray audibly, but I sat down by his bed and shut my teeth, and I said in my soul, "Now, Mr. Devil, go to it. You kill him if you can." And I sat there five days and nights. He did not get healing instantly the second time. It was healing by process. Because of that fact, my soul took hold on God; I sat with my teeth shut, and I never left his bedside until it was done.

You may be healed like a sunburst of God today, and tomorrow, the next week, or the next month when you want healing, you may have to take it on the slow process. The action of God is not always the same, because the conditions are not always the same.

In the life of Jesus, people were instantly healed. I believe Jesus has such a supreme measure of the Spirit that when He put His hands on a man, he was filled and submerged in the Holy Ghost, and the diseases withered out and vanished.

But, beloved, you and I use the measure of the Spirit that we possess. (You can, as a member of His body, possess the Spirit in the same measure as He; God does not expect us to fulfill John 14:12 with less equipment than Jesus had.) And if we haven't got as much of God as Jesus had, then you pray for a man today, and you get a certain measure of healing, but he is not entirely well. The only thing to do is to pray for him tomorrow, and let him get some more, and keep on until he is well.

That is where people blunder. They will pray for a day or two, and then they quit. You pray and keep on day by day and minister to your sick until they are well. One of the things that has discredited healing is that evangelists will hold meetings, and hundreds of sick will come and be prayed for. In a great meeting like that, you get a chance to pray once and do not see them again. You pray for ten people, and as a rule, you will find that one or two or three are absolutely healed, but the others are only half-healed or quarter-healed or have only a little touch of healing.

It is just the same with salvation. You bring ten to the altar. One is saved and is clear in his soul. Another may come for a week, and another for a month, before they are clear in their souls. The difference is not with God. The difference is inside the man. His consciousness has not opened up to God.

Every law of the Spirit that applies to salvation applies to healing likewise.

And when Jesus was entered into Capernaum, there came unto him a centurion, beseeching him, and saying, Lord, my servant lieth at home sick of the palsy, grievously tormented. And Jesus saith unto him, I will come and heal him. The centurion answered and said, Lord, I am not

worthy that thou shouldest come under my roof: but speak the word only,
and my servant shall be healed.   (Matthew 8:5–8)

Here is healing at a distance. That centurion understood divine authority, and the same divine authority is vested in the Christian, for Jesus is the
pattern Christian.

For I am a man under authority, having soldiers under me: and I say to
this man, Go, and he goeth; and to another, Come, and he cometh; and
to my servant, Do this, and he doeth it.   (Matthew 8:9)

The same divine authority that was vested in Jesus is vested by Jesus in
every Christian soul. Jesus made provision for the church of Jesus Christ to
go on forever and do the same things as He did and to keep on doing them
forever. That is what is the matter with the church. The church has lost faith
in that truth. The result, they went on believing He could save them from sin,
but the other great range of Christian life was left to the doctors and the devil
or anything else. And the church will never be a real church, in the real power
of the living God again, until she comes back again to the original standard,
where Jesus was.

Jesus said, "Behold, I give you authority." What authority? *"Against*
unclean spirits, to cast them out, and to heal all manner of sickness and all manner
of disease" (Matthew 10:1). Jesus has vested that authority in you. You say,
"Well Lord, we understand the authority that is in your Word, but we haven't
the power." But Jesus said, *"Ye shall receive power, after that the Holy Ghost is*
come upon you" (Acts 1:8).

Now the Holy Ghost is come upon every Christian in a measure. It is a
question of degree! There are degrees of the measure of the Spirit of God in
men's lives. The *baptism of the Holy Spirit* is a greater measure of the Spirit of
God, but every man has a degree of the Holy Spirit in his life. You have. It is
the Spirit in your life that gives you faith in God, that makes you a blessing to
other people. It is the Holy Spirit that is *outbreathed* in your soul that touches
another soul and moves them for God. Begin right where you are and let God
take you along the Christian life as far as you like.

When Jesus heard it, he marveled, and said to them that followed, Verily
I say unto you, I have not found so great faith, no, not in Israel.
(Matthew 8:10)

Jesus always commended faith when He met it. Jesus did not always meet faith. All the people who came to Jesus did not possess that order of faith. They had faith that if they got to Jesus, they would be healed. But here was a man who said, *"Speak the word only, and my servant shall be healed"* (Matthew 8:8).

Then you remember the case of the man at the pool of Bethesda. He did not even ask to be healed. As he lay there, Jesus walked up to him and said, *"Wilt thou be made whole?"* (John 5:6). He saw this poor chap who had been lying there for thirty-eight years, and Jesus did not wait for him to ask Him to heal. Jesus said, *"Wilt thou be made whole?"* and the poor fellow went on to say that when the water was troubled, he had no one to put him in, but while he was waiting another stepped in ahead of him. But Jesus said to him, *"Rise, take up thy bed, and walk"* (John 5:8). He was made whole. Afterward, Jesus met him and said, *"Behold, thou art made whole: sin no more, lest a worse thing come unto thee"* (verse 14).

Most of sickness is the result of sin. That is the answer to the individual who sins. For thousands of years men have been sinning, and in consequence of their sin, they are diseased in their bodies. This will give you an idea. Scientists tell us there are tubercular germs in 90 percent of the population. The only difference is that when people keep in a healthy state, the germs do not get a chance to manifest themselves. I am trying to show the intimacy between sin and sickness, not necessarily the sin of the individual. It may never be the sin of the individual.

In records of the Lake and Graham family away back, tuberculosis was never known to them, until it appeared in my sister. My sister accompanied me to Africa, and she became so ill that when I got to Cape Town, we had to wait until her strength returned. God healed her.

Regarding people being healed at a distance, we receive telegrams from all over the world. Distance is no barrier to God. The United States has just finished the building of the greatest wireless station in the world. They send messages that register almost instantly across ten thousand miles. When the machine is touched here, it registers ten thousand miles away. Well, all right, when your *heart* strikes God in faith, it will register wherever that individual is, just that quick. All the discoveries of later years such as telegraph, telephone, wireless, and that sort of thing are just the common laws that Christians have practiced all their lives.

Nobody ever knelt down and prayed, but that the instant he touched God, his soul registered in Jesus Christ in glory, and the answer came back to the soul. Christians have that experience every day. The wise world has begun to observe that these laws are applicable in the natural realm. I asked Marconi once how he got his first idea for the wireless. He replied that he got it from watching an exhibition of telepathy in a cheap theater.

The prayer of the heart reaches God. Jesus replied to the leper, "*I will*; be clean." The next was the centurion's servant. The centurion said, "You do not need to come to my house. You *speak the word only*, and my servant shall be healed," and in His soul, Jesus said, "Be healed." Distance is no barrier to God. Distance makes no difference. The Spirit of God in you will go as far as your love reaches. *Love* is the medium that conveys the Spirit of God to another soul anywhere on God's earth.

This is what takes place as you pray. The Spirit of God comes upon you and bathes your soul, and a shaft of it reaches out and touches that soul over there. If you had an instrument that was fine enough to photograph spirit, you would discover this is done.

Is it not a marvelous thing that God has chosen us to be co-laborers with Him and that He takes us into partnership to do all that He is doing? Jesus Christ at the throne of God desires the blessing of you and me, and out of His holy heart the Spirit comes, and the soul is filled, and we cannot tell how or why.

I have known thousands of people to be healed who have never seen my face. They send a request for prayer, we pray, and we never hear anything more about them sometimes unless a friend or a neighbor or someone comes and tells us about them. Sometimes someone sends in a request for them. They will tell you they do not know what happened. They just got well. But you know why. That is the wonderful power there is in the Christian life, and that is the wonderful cooperation that the Lord Jesus has arranged between

His own soul and the soul of the Christian. That is *"the church, which is his body"* (Ephesians 1:22–23).

Jesus came to *"destroy the works of the devil"* (1 John 3:8). He healed all that were oppressed of the devil. (See Acts 10:38.) He did not use carnal weapons in destroying the work of the devil. He used a spiritual weapon. It is best expressed in Luke:

> *And the whole multitude sought to touch him: for there went virtue [power] out of him, and healed them all.* (Luke 6:19)

This is the perfect remedy for all of man's ills. Jesus taught His disciples the use of this weapon. He sent out the twelve, and He sent out the seventy. (See Luke 9:1–2; 10:1–19.) That His training was not fruitless is shown by the book of the Acts of the Apostles. Acting in the name of Jesus, the outflow of power from their lives brought healing to all who came to them. They duplicated His ministry. There is not one record of a failure in the book of Acts. The weapons of their warfare against the work of the devil in forms of sickness and disease were spiritual and not carnal. (See 2 Corinthians 10:4.) The same power is available today.

> *Behold, I give unto you power to tread on serpents and scorpions, and over all the power of the enemy: and nothing shall by any means hurt you.* (Luke 10:19)

God gives the members of the body of His Son power over the devil. He never gives the devil power over them.

One of the marvels of Christianity is the power given the believer. *"Resist the devil, and he will flee from you"* (James 4:7). The devil cannot make a believer do a single thing without the believer's consent or assent. Resist the devil and he flees. Give in and he wins. It is this fact, as simple as it may sound, that constitutes our responsibility for our behavior. So that no person can say, "I sinned in spite of myself," but he or she can only say, "I sinned because of myself."

Cleansed from all sin (root, stem, and branch) so that the devil has no anchor within and having put on the invincible armor of Ephesians 6, the believer is the master in every situation. If the believer stands firm and uses his armor efficiently, he is unbeatable by the devil.

Couple all that is said above with this statement from 1 John 4:4: *"Greater is he that is in you, than he that is in the world"*—why then should a believer ever give in to the devil and sin?

I can identify with Jesus as a member of His body when He said, *"The prince of this world cometh, and hath nothing in me"* (John 14:30). Why let the devil in or put anything in?

"And the God of peace shall bruise [shatter completely] Satan under your feet shortly" (Romans 16:20). In any warfare there comes a time when the enemy is shattered. Stand true and allow God to shatter him under your feet. Stand fast!

Journey into Word & Spirit

1. Do you believe that you need someone to lay hands on you to be healed? Or is your faith such that you can say right now to the Lord, *"Speak the word only, and [Your] servant shall be healed"* (Matthew 8:8)?

2. If you still feel undeserving of the Lord's healing touch, what is holding you back?

Chapter excerpted from Roberts Liardon, comp., *John G. Lake on Healing* (New Kensington, PA: Whitaker House, 2009), chapter 11, "Behold, I Give You Power."

About the Author

John Graham Lake (1870–1935) was a businessman who became known for his ministry as a missionary, faith healer, and founder of the Apostolic Faith Mission of South Africa. He was influenced by the healing ministry of John Alexander Dowie, and he received the baptism of the Holy Spirit in 1907 in the wake of the Azusa Street Revival. Lake moved to Spokane, Washington, in September 1914. He began ministering in The Church of Truth. After six months, he opened his own building, which he called Lake's Divine Healing Rooms. He began training "Divine Healing Technicians" in an organization he founded called The Divine Healing Institute. From February 1915 until May 1920, Lake and his DHTs reported over 100,000 healings.

HOW TO TOUCH THE LORD

Kathryn Kuhlman

14

HOW TO TOUCH THE LORD

Kathryn Kuhlman

Those who know me are aware of my great respect for doctors and their vast medical and scientific knowledge; and without any desire or thought to belittle their sincere efforts, let it be said that God can and will do what no man can do in healing ALL who will come to Him by faith in the name of His Son. He is no respecter of persons.

The power of God will become real to your heart in a beautiful way when He touches your body and the healing virtue of Jesus Christ flows through you. It will enhance the spiritual blessings which you may have enjoyed for a long time. It will enrich your testimony. It will enable you to encourage others who stand in great need. It will challenge the unsaved, and may well be the means of leading others to a saving knowledge of the Lord Jesus Christ, by far the greatest miracle of all.

Since God, His Son Jesus, and the Holy Spirit are supernatural, it is natural that we should expect God to do supernatural things for us. We can live in the state of expectancy that He will perform miracles, and among them are miracles of healing for our physical bodies, healing all who will reach out and touch the hem of His garment, all who will say, "Jesus, You are all You claim to be."

The place that the Word of God needs to occupy has been yielded to tradition. Doubt has robbed many of us of the rewards that result when we believe God's promises. Opinions have usurped the seat of God's positive declarations. God's people have become eloquent in excuses, allowing an almost total lack of evidence of a living Christ in their lives. Jesus is as willing to heal today as He was when a leper cried out to Him: *"Lord, if thou wilt, thou canst make me clean. And Jesus put forth his hand, and touched him, saying, I will; be thou clean. And immediately his leprosy was cleansed"* (Matthew 8:2–3).

⌣

The Healing Virtue

The healing virtue, or power, that Jesus uses is the Holy Spirit, the Third Person of the Godhead. To understand something of His personality and His work will make it easier for you to bring belief to the stature of faith.

Let this simple statement sink into the very deepest recesses of your heart. *The Holy Spirit can and will do anything and everything for you that Jesus Himself would were He standing there before you with His hands extended and the radiant light of glory shining from His face.* In fact, Jesus sent the Holy Spirit when He went to be with the Father: *"I will pray the Father, and he shall give you another Comforter, that he may abide with you for ever"* (John 14:16).

That glorious promise in John 14:16 says several startling things. It shows the three members of the Godhead in divine harmony of action. It reveals that the Holy Spirit will be *"another"* like unto Himself, a Comforter, a Strengthener. It shows that the Holy Spirit will continue and abide *"for ever."*

Instead of the Great Physician having limitations of the flesh, accessible to a relatively small number, He becomes accessible to ALL of us through the Holy Spirit. The Great Physician is everywhere today. He is all-sufficient, for Jesus not only has power in heaven, but all power in earth as well.

This fact alone should be enough to change our entire outlook. It is not merely a matter of getting something from God, as important as that may be to you. It is a matter of "practicing the presence of God," of recognizing, enjoying, and utilizing the continual abiding presence of the Holy Spirit.

Remember that the Holy Spirit is with you whether you think so or not, whether you feel His presence or are wholly unaware of it. If you are a true child of God, then you have the witness of the Holy Spirit which is your assurance of salvation. This Holy Spirit is the same one who worked with Jesus during His earthly ministry in the performance of His healing miracles.

To understand that enables you to see what great power there is available to you now. It is the same as when Jesus walked the shores of Galilee. The only difference is that you have MORE on which to base your faith, for His testimony has been established and corroborated thousands of times and more since then.

When Lydia touched the hem of the Lord's garment, the Word declares: *"And Jesus, immediately knowing in himself that virtue had gone out of him, turned him about in the press, and said, Who touched my clothes?"* (Mark 5:30).

The virtue that *"had gone out of him"* was the power of the Holy Spirit flowing through His very being. It did not mean that He had any the less of that power because He had been touched by Lydia, but that another through Him had received of it.

One ordinarily thinks of virtue as being a "specific kind of goodness" or characteristic. That is true. The kind of goodness in this instance is the divine nature, the perfection, the holiness and righteousness of Almighty God. This is one point on which many fail in their understanding of how God works in the healing of the body, or in answering prayer for any benefit or blessing. They fail to see that they are asking God to touch them with the high zenith of absolute purity, the power of perfect holiness. That is His virtue.

We should realize, therefore, that this requires prayerful consideration; that sincere, earnest, honest heart cleansing should precede any request of the Lord to exercise this virtue for our benefit. Far better that we come to Him pleading His mercy, "Lord, cleanse my heart with the precious blood of the Lamb. Make me pure and clean from all my sin. Make my heart right in the sight of God," than to come with the attitude that He must heal us in spite of the sinful condition of our lives, or without any desire on our part to serve Him, or to render Him glory in testimony after He does heal us. Remember, you ask for a part of God when you ask Him to give of His virtue and His power.

In other words, remember to come unto the Lord with all the heart warmth and utter reverence that you would feel if you were to suddenly find yourself confronted by the Person of the Son of God, for the Holy Spirit is God in exactly the same way as Jesus is God, and as the Father is God.

Jesus Christ now sits at the right hand of God the Father in glory. He still has the body of Calvary and bears the scars of the crucifixion. He is our Savior, and He is in position of great High Priest.

The Holy Spirit is here. He is with us now. We can feel His presence, practice His presence, utilize His presence, praise God in His presence, and live under the blood of Jesus in His presence.

Let it be said that this healing virtue is obtained through Christ and in no other way. All that is done by the Holy Spirit is done in the name of Jesus, and the Holy Spirit will definitely lead you to give Jesus all the glory for your healing after He has touched you. The Holy Spirit is carrying out the injunction of Jesus when He is with you, when He blesses you, when He keeps you, when He heals you. Remember that Jesus sent the Holy Spirit when He returned to the Father in Heaven.

Lest someone feel that the work of healing sick bodies is given precedence over the greater ministry of the Holy Spirit in bringing conviction and conversion to the unsaved, it must be pointed out in this connection that the same power that heals sick bodies also convicts and saves. There is but one Holy Spirit, and whenever and wherever He is present for healing the sick, He is also present in revival power. In fact, many great revivals have resulted from the performance of healing miracles. That was true in the Lord's ministry to such an extent that He even told that He was healing so that they might believe also for salvation.

Church members today need to stop limiting the ministry of the Holy Spirit, and begin praying and believing God for the enriching and enlarging work of the Third Person of the Trinity in His blessed fullness. Jesus meant the Holy Spirit to be as Himself among us until the very end of this age, which will close when He returns at the Catching Up.

The "touch of the Lord" is the moving of the Holy Spirit in us, through us, and for us. He will supply any and every need in your life when you will simply believe God.

How to Touch the Lord

In Mark's account of the healing of Lydia, she is referred to as a *"certain woman"* (Mark 5:25), and so also are you a certain man or a certain woman in the sight of the Lord today. It is as though you are the only person in all the world in need of His touch, and though you may be in a vast multitude, God will single you out if you touch Him by faith.

Matthew records that Lydia *"said within herself, If I may but touch his garment, I shall be whole"* (Matthew 9:21). Her discussion and persuasion were within her own heart. She knew in herself that Jesus would heal her, and so she was healed. This is how to "touch" the Lord: be absolutely persuaded in your own heart that He will meet your need.

Lydia had an urgent need of the Lord's help. That need was so great that all lesser things were relegated to lesser places of importance in her consideration. Her consuming thought was for the healing of her body. She was desperate about the matter. She did not approach the Lord with the idea that IF He healed her, it would be wonderful; and that IF He did not heal her, she would not be too much surprised or disappointed. Her need was far too great for that. She already knew that, medically speaking, there was no help. She went to Jesus with her whole heart and mind as well as with her sick body. That is how to touch the Lord: with a whole heart and a mind single to His performing the need of the hour.

Lydia had no other hope. It was Jesus and Jesus only who held the answer to her dilemma, and those of us who reach that place in the concentration of our need and our faith will surely know the Lord's healing touch.

Sometimes it is not easy to reach the Lord, for there are obstacles such as Lydia knew. There was her weakness to be considered. Her strength and her life's blood were far spent. Besides, hundreds of people were milling about

Jesus, each seeking for himself a better view, a clearer hearing, or a gratification of his own curiosity or heart hunger. People often stand in the way when one is trying to get closer to Jesus, close enough to reach out and touch Him. Most often they are well meaning people, but we fear what they will think or what they will say. Instead, we need to be encouraged to trust the Lord, and this assurance is many times found on our knees in prayer.

Press through, beloved, press through! No matter who may stand in the way, press through. You need not explain or make your determination audible, just simply and persistently press through to Jesus. Lydia made a desperate effort to reach her Lord, and He was there to honor her faith and to meet her need. She merely touched the hem of the Master's robe. She did not handle Him, she did not tug at Him, she touched His garment; but that was enough. This started the mighty power of the Holy Spirit coursing through her body and made her well and whole again. No, Lydia was not worthy to touch Jesus (and neither are we); yet, she knew that He forgave sins when He healed, and that He healed all manner of sickness and disease. She knew He had never turned anyone away who came to Him, and she knew to reverence Him as the Holy One, the Son of the Living God.

The Prayer of Faith

The true prayer of faith may be just that and nothing more. It would seem from the record that Jairus' word to Jesus was that kind of prayer: *"My little daughter lieth at the point of death: I pray thee, come and lay thy hands on her, that she may be healed; and she shall live"* (Mark 5:23). Of course Jesus went, and even though the little child had died before He reached her bedside, she was raised up by the power of God. No matter what the need, Jairus saw Jesus ready, willing, and able to heal.

The prayer of faith is in reality the heart act of receiving that which we ask the Lord to do. *"Now faith is the substance of things hoped for..."* (Hebrews 11:1). *"Believe that ye receive [it]"* (Mark 11:24). It is not the mere act of petitioning the Lord and certainly not the condition of begging. It is the heart act of receiving from the Lord with the positive knowledge that the material evidences are to be made known at His pleasure, for your good, and for His glory.

Perhaps you are saying at this point, "I would give anything in the world for a faith like that"; but do not start trying to measure your faith to see how great or how small it is. By the time you are finished, you may likely seem to have no faith at all. Don't try to "take your faith out" and look at it. Your faith is the result, at any given time, of your heart relation to Jesus. Surely you have experienced moments when you have exercised great faith, and other times when you feel your faith is small. Begin your season of petitioning with consecration, with praise, with worship…*"Be careful for nothing; but in every thing by prayer and supplication with* **thanksgiving** *let your requests be made known unto God"* (Philippians 4:6).

The prayer of faith is not the result of having used a measuring rod to find a level on your state of belief at a given moment. Neither is the fact that at one time you received a mighty answer to prayer, definite proof that you have faith now; nor the fact that you never had an acknowledged answer to prayer, any reason to believe that you cannot pray the prayer of faith today.

Your faith is the result of your heart relation to Jesus. Surely there are times when you will exercise great faith and other times when you feel that you have little faith. This is why the prescribed formula begins with praise, worship, consecration, [and] thankfulness for past favors and blessings. This is why faith is great when a spiritual revival is in progress; why God's child, awed by the beauty of Jesus, the surety of the Word, the goodness of the Father, and the sweet presence of the Spirit, can easily believe for anything and everything.

The prayer of faith, then, should be the experience of every believer, enriching his testimony, making joyous his heart, and a source of praise to Him who hears and answers prayer.

Journey into Word & Spirit

1. How is God calling you to "touch the hem of His garment"? Is there something specific He is asking you to do in pursuit of healing?

2. Ask the Lord for a gift of faith. Search the Scriptures and ask God to reveal truths about this gift of faith. What do you already know about it?

3. Spend some time worshipping the Lord and thanking Him for His presence, love, and faithfulness. Ask Him to allow you to tangibly experience His presence filling you. Can you feel His healing touch?

Chapter excerpted from Kathryn Kuhlman, *The Lord's Healing Touch* (Pittsburgh, PA: The Kathryn Kuhlman Foundation, 1960), 133–149.

About the Author

Kathryn Kuhlman was a well-known evangelist who held miracle services throughout the United States. On July 4, 1948, she launched her first miracle service at Carnegie Hall in Pittsburgh, Pennsylvania. Through the decades, she became a popular evangelist—especially after she expanded her reach into media and moved from radio to television with her program *I Believe in Miracles.* Through her television show and her meetings, thousands of people came to salvation and experienced healing. For more information on Kathryn Kuhlman, visit www.kathrynkuhlman.com.

THE KINGDOM OF POWER

Guillermo Maldonado

15

THE KINGDOM OF POWER

Guillermo Maldonado

Faith is to the kingdom of God what currency is for a nation. In today's society, the strongest currencies in the world are losing their strength, people's purchasing power is fluctuating, and most people do not feel financially secure. Only the kingdom of God is unshakable. Its currency is always strong, and it allows us to acquire everything we need from the eternal realm. However, if we are to receive from what is in eternity, we must understand what faith is, how it functions, and how to walk according to it.

What Is Faith?

After studying Hebrews 11:1 comprehensively, I developed the following as a summation of what I believe is its essential meaning:

Now, faith is; and it is the reality of the main foundation on which hope rests, the conviction of all that truly exists and the controller of the things we do not see.

Let me expound on this statement according to its various parts, as we… explore the question "What is faith?"

1. "Now…"

Man has placed in the future what God has placed in the present. In the mind and realm of God, the present and the future exist together, and faith is the currency with which we obtain the future *now*. I don't believe He ever wanted there to be a delay between the will of heaven and the manifestation of that will of earth—"*Your kingdom come. Your will be done on earth as it is in heaven*" (Matthew 6:10 NKJV). God did not "try" to create light on earth by saying, a hundred times, "*Let there be light…*" (Genesis 1:3 NKJV). He said it once, and there was light.

Through faith, we enter into the "time zone"
of the kingdom in the "now" of God.

When Jesus manifested the supernatural, His faith worked according to the leading of the Holy Spirit and the rhema of God for that moment. (See Matthew 4:4.) He said,

> *The Son can do nothing of Himself, but what He sees the Father do; for whatever He does, the Son also does in like manner.* (John 5:19 NKJV)

In the same way, we must daily rely on God to show us what He is doing in heaven so that we can do it on earth. (See Romans 8:14.) This is how we receive immediate manifestations from the eternal realm and avoid getting into trouble by trying to declare something on our own. Notice that when Christ ministered on earth, there was no delay between His declared word and its manifestation. We see examples of this reality in the deliverance of the Syro-Phoenician woman's daughter (see Mark 7:29–30), the deliverance of the demon-possessed man (see Mark 9:25–27), the calming of the storm at sea (see Mark 4:38–39), and the resurrection of Lazarus (see John 11:43–44).

Christ operated in the revealed faith of the here and now.
Every miracle He did was in the now.

Jesus did not confess a hundred times, "Lazarus, come out!" He called Lazarus once, and a man who had been dead for four days came out of his tomb alive. Jesus had received a rhema from the Holy Spirit pertaining to that situation and the time when Lazarus would resurrect. Note also that Jesus never prayed for the sick or the demon possessed when He cured them—nowhere in the Bible does it say that He prayed for them. Neither did He say to anyone, "You will be healed sometime in the near future." Rather, Jesus declared the sick healed, and they were healed! He simply made declarations, such as *"Be healed of your affliction"* (Mark 5:34 NKJV), *"Rise, take up your bed and walk"* (John 5:8 NKJV), and *"Your faith has made you well"* (see, for example, Luke 18:42 NKJV). Likewise, He cast out demons, and they immediately fled!

Jesus spoke based on the truth rather than the facts as they appeared in the natural world. Every miracle He performed came to pass because He spoke with faith from the eternal realm as a result of a revealed word in the present. If Jesus Christ did this, we can do it, also. (See John 14:12.) Read through the book of Acts, and you will see that there was no lapse of time between the apostles' declarations and the visible manifestations of God's power. In my own ministry, the most powerful miracles I have witnessed have taken place the moment the word left my mouth. We will witness the most extraordinary miracles of all time when we receive and practice the revelation that faith is now. As our old mind-set is renewed, everything we say, decree, declare, and pray will no longer be for the future but in the now.

In Christ, all things are in the now. Outside of Him,
all things are subject to time.

Melina García of Colombia had suffered from alopecia areata (hair loss) since she was twelve years old. The doctors could not find the underlying cause or a cure. They thought her condition might have been triggered by stress or a vitamin deficiency, but no corresponding treatment worked. She lost a significant amount of hair every time she combed it. People would stare at her, and this made her uncomfortable, so she would attempt to arrange her hair to hide the bald spots. Her condition had caused her self-esteem to plummet.

Melina then attended CAP (Apostolic and Prophetic Conference) Colombia, sponsored by King Jesus Ministry, and she prayed for a miracle. During one of the sessions, as I declared healing over different illnesses, the Holy Spirit led me to decree that hair was growing on people who were bald. Instantly, Melina felt a supernatural weight come upon her, and she fell to the floor. When she got up, she checked her head and felt new hair! Every place where there had been a bald spot was now covered! She went back to the doctor, who could not explain what had happened. Her miracle was not for the future but in the now.

The future is the eternal present postponed.

I witness miracles like Melina's everywhere I go, and the entire church of Jesus Christ can witness similar miracles multiplied many times over as we expand the kingdom of God on the earth. The only condition is that we constantly exercise the measure of faith God has given us. When we do this, our faith will increase exponentially, because the more we use our faith, the more faith we will be given.

> *I am God, and there is none like Me, declaring the end from the beginning.* (Isaiah 46:9–10 NKJV)

Many of us have been trained to pray and then wait an indeterminate amount of time until something happens, but God is the God of the here and now. He declares *"the end from the beginning."* So, if we declare that something will take place in a week, a month, or a year, we delay its manifestation or materialization in the present. When we believe miracles "will" take place, "sometime," they are like an airplane stuck in a circling pattern over an airport, unable to land. However, we can remove all delays when we live in the now, so that the miracles can "land," and we can receive them.

People often prefer to believe for healing rather than for miracles, because healing is usually progressive (see, for example, Mark 16:18) and demands less risk to our faith. In contrast, miracles take place instantly, so they require an immediate response from those receiving them. If we don't respond instantly, we may lose them. Some blessings in our lives are being detained because we have established a future due date for their arrival. When we combine a rhema with "now" faith, we can receive them today.

Faith takes something from the eternal "future" and materializes it in the present.

2. "Faith Is…"

Before we were born on earth, we existed in eternity. In God, we first "are" in the spiritual realm, and then we manifest in the physical realm. This is because God determines the purpose for something before He creates it, and He finishes everything before He starts it. Our job is to discover what "is" in God's eternal realm so that we can bring it into our physical realm through faith.

In Western culture, most people reverse this process. Rather than starting with who they are, they "do" things to try to gain acceptance by others, so that they can "be" someone. This is how people become slaves to public opinion and never really know who they were born to be.

The Scripture says,

For as [a person] *thinks in his heart, so is he.*   (Proverbs 23:7 NKJV)

To operate in the kingdom of God, we begin with who we "are" in eternity. When we know that we are God's beloved children, chosen from the foundation of the world (see Ephesians 1:4), and discover who He created us to be, we will think and act from that perspective. Everything else will develop from our identity and existence in Him. Our "being" will lead to our "doing," and not the other way around. We will not aspire to "become" something, because we already "are"!

You are a child of God with a unique purpose; and because you are in Christ, you receive every spiritual blessing in Him. (See Ephesians 1:3.) God designed you to be saved, righteous, holy, at peace, joyful, blessed, healthy, free, prosperous, and more. You don't have to wait for someday in the future to be saved, healed, prosperous, and so forth, because you "are" those things! Receive them now!

Faith enables us to remain in the state of
"being" supernatural, in the now.

---

3. *"The Reality of the Main Foundation on Which Hope Rests…"*

The above phrase reflects the following portion of Hebrews 11:1 (NKJV): "the substance of things hoped for…." The Greek word translated "substance" is hupostasis, which means "a setting under (support)." In a figurative sense, it means "essence," or "assurance." Among its other indications are "confidence" and "substance" (STRONG, G5287).

Basically, to exercise faith means to "sit upon" the Word that God gave us; to rest on it, or submit to it, knowing that God will keep it. When we rest, we are in faith. When we worry, we are not in faith; as a result, our hope—in the sense of confident expectation—has no substance. Faith is the assurance that what we believe is real and legally ours. No one can have a legal deed to a nonexistent property. Faith is the authentic or reliable proof that guarantees the existence of what we believe for. Even though we have yet to see it with our natural eyes, it is a reality, because has God promised it.

Faith "is," and we do not hope for something that "is" but something that will be. (See Romans 8:24–25.) Hope is for the realm of time, but faith is for now. If salvation, healing, and deliverance exist now, then why are we still waiting for them? To wait is to apply hope to matters where faith should be in operation. For example, hope enables us to wait for the second coming of

Christ in His glory, but faith enables us to expect and receive health, salvation, prosperity, and miracles in the here and now.

Faith acts and stands on what God has already predetermined, generating expectation.

God is releasing supernatural expectation in believers. During a leaders' conference in Argentina, I met Oliver Inchausti, a seven-year-old who had been deaf in his right ear since birth because the ear had not developed properly and was deformed, having no orifice. Oliver's deafness considerably affected his ability to interact with his surroundings and to develop language skills. His mother had consulted many doctors, who gave a variety of advice. Some said they didn't even know if Oliver really had an eardrum, because it was very small. One specialist suggested that she take him to Cuba for surgery. Brazilian doctors said they could do surgery that would enable him to hear through his bone. Other plastic surgeons said they could do nothing until he became an adult.

When Oliver and his mother attended the leaders' conference, they came to the altar when I called all those who were deaf to come and demonstrate faith in the now. This young boy had spent years yearning for a miracle, so he was expecting something to happen. I placed my hand on his deaf ear and declared the miracle. His mother then placed her hand over his good ear, and one of my doctors tested him from behind his deaf ear. As soon as the doctor said a word, Oliver repeated it clearly and without hesitation. He heard perfectly! The doctor examined his ear and saw that the small orifice had increased in size.

Can you imagine what would happen if an entire congregation expected to receive something from God? In my ministry travels, I often experience the demand of faith upon the mantle of miracles God has given me from people who have great expectations. When this happens, miracles, signs, and wonders are released among them.

⌣

How to Live and Move in "Now" Faith

If you are at a standstill in your faith, it means you have done everything within your own power or knowledge but have run out of your own resources. You need new resources, which God is providing today. Step by step, you can go "*from faith to faith*" (Romans 1:17 NKJV). God wants to move you into the dimension of faith that is in the here and now—for miracles, signs, wonders, and acceleration in the advancement of His kingdom.

What I am about to teach you are principles and revelations I have observed and experienced over the course of twenty-plus years in ministry. If you believe them and put them into practice, I promise that you will do the same things that I have been doing, and even greater things. Walking, living, and moving in "now" faith requires [several steps, including] the following...:

Operate Your Faith from a Place of Righteousness

> *Behold the proud, his soul is not upright in him; but the just shall live by his faith.* (Habakkuk 2:4 NKJV)

We were saved and justified by faith, and it is only by faith that we can live and function in God's kingdom. Righteousness is the foundation of faith. We may have faith to believe and to declare a manifestation from the eternal realm, but if we are not right with God in any area of our lives, our faith can be nullified. For example, if we don't tithe or give offerings to God, our faith for finances or a job will not work, even if we believe with great zeal, because we are robbing God. We won't have access to the benefits that God has promised to those who tithe. In the family, if one spouse abuses the other, his or her faith becomes ineffective. (See 1 Peter 3:7.)

This principle is applicable in every area of our lives and ministry. Even though God wants to back up our belief and declarations, He is unable to do so because it would mean going against His Word and righteousness.

Does the kingdom of darkness know when we are not walking in righteousness? Of course, it does! Demons know when we are not exercising our faith properly, because they live in the spirit realm and are aware when our faith has substance and when it lacks the integrity of righteousness. We should pause right now and ask ourselves if there is unrighteousness in any area of our lives. If so, we must repent and allow the blood of Jesus to cleanse us. This will activate the righteousness of the kingdom in us, and God will be able to bless us according to His promises.

The law of righteousness makes faith operative; unrighteousness makes it inoperative.

Walk by Faith, Not by Sight

For we walk by faith, not by sight. (2 Corinthians 5:7 NKJV)

"*Sight*" represents the limitations of our natural environment, surroundings, circumstances, difficulties, obstacles, sicknesses, lack, impossibilities, and more. Such things are the opposite of faith. In order to rise above them, we must acquire a different perspective and reality. If our thoughts are consumed by a hard situation, problem, or obstacle, we are not living by faith. The natural world is unstable, insecure, and temporal, but God does not change. When we walk by faith and not sight, our reality no longer depends on our environment or circumstances but on His eternal reality, and we become everything He has called us to be.

Everything that is not eternal is subject to change.

Some people walk according to a "neutral optimism" rather than by faith. For example, they say, "If a miracle happens, it is God's will, but if it doesn't happen, it is not His will." Jesus did not preach or act according to this mindset, but much of the church seems to have adopted it, thus conforming to a "probability" mentality. If we pray for healing but nothing happens, that's okay; if we pray for provision and nothing happens, that's okay, too. This detached attitude reveals our apathy and demonstrates our lack of expectation to receive from God.

Other people walk according to trust instead of faith. Sometimes, these terms are used interchangeably. However, trust is generally a feeling that operates in relationships, whereas faith is a heavenly substance that operates in the spirit realm and doesn't depend on emotions or circumstances. Trust works on the basis of our mental knowledge and emotional experience of a person's prior faithfulness and competence, but faith operates on the basis of revelation knowledge in the now, given by the Holy Spirit to our spirits. Therefore, in spiritual matters, our trust will not operate beyond what we personally know and have experienced of God. It won't lead us to believe in what we have not yet received from Him. It takes faith to move from what we have already seen, heard, or felt to what is newly revealed by the Holy Spirit.

Faith is a continuous, supernatural walk with God in the now.

Decide right now to rise above the places, people, and things that keep you from walking and growing in faith. Begin to edify a new atmosphere of faith in your life and home. Do not conform to the temporal; enter the spirit realm, where faith can change your reality. Sickness, problems, adversity, and trials were never ordained to be permanent. Yet we have learned to tolerate them, and we have turned them into something permanent by saying, "*My* sickness; *my* cancer; *my* pain; *my* lack; *my* depression…." We speak of these things as if they belonged to us, but they don't! Rebuke them right now!

Everything to which we conform will become
our reality and mind-set.

Rise Above Human Reason Through the Spirit and the Word

The things that are possible in heaven are rejected by human reason because they are outside our natural experience. We will not find faith until we rise above reason, because God will continually ask us to do things that do not make sense to our finite intellect. Miracles, signs, and wonders go beyond the ability of our natural mind to comprehend because their purpose is to demonstrate and manifest the supernatural.

If we use reason to evaluate an illness, situation, adversity, or calamity, it could turn deadly. What does a doctor usually do when explaining to a patient that he has a fatal illness? He tries to convince the patient to own the sickness and to make the best of it, because nothing else can be done. The doctor may have the best intentions toward the patient, but he is weakening that person's faith. If the doctor tells someone he has only a short time left to live, the patient's faith is the only thing that can break that word, because faith is able to enter eternity and pull from it whatever he needs in the now. I appreciate doctors and medicine; they are useful to humanity. I also know that sickness is a fact. I don't tell people to negate the facts, but I affirm that there are eternal truths, such as divine healing, that are above temporal facts, such as sickness.

The truth that exists above the reality presented by the doctor is that Jesus' death on the cross provided for our healing. Knowing this, we must decide whom we will believe. Will we believe the doctor or God? The diagnosis or His Word? Sickness or faith?

Faith is the ability to believe what reason finds nonsensical.

The Holy Spirit enables us to rise above our reason and common sense. When we receive the baptism of the Holy Spirit, we are given the gift of speaking in spiritual tongues, or languages, not understood by our reason. (See, for example, Acts 10:44–47; 1 Corinthians 14:2.) God gave us tongues to enable us to bypass our minds so that we could communicate with Him and receive from Him in the spiritual realm. If you have not yet been baptized with the Spirit, ask God to give you this gift of His supernatural power and presence. Then, stop paying attention to circumstances and begin to declare and obey, by faith, the rhema you receive from the Spirit. Also, don't lose the blessing just because it may be hard to understand. Understanding is not a requirement for obeying God, and living by faith always entails an element of risk.

Correspondingly, our reality should be determined by the truth—the Word of God—which operates beyond human reason as the highest level of reality. My job as a teacher of the Word includes dealing with people's disbelief as they try to "reason things out." I work alongside the Holy Spirit and the truth of the Scriptures to demonstrate to people that their reason makes no sense according to the laws of the supernatural realm. As their spiritual eyes are opened, they set aside reason and fill the void with the logic of God. The supernatural begins to make sense to them, because they see from His point of view.

Pastor David Alcántara of Honduras, one of my spiritual sons, reported that "a man named Manuel, who is a chauffeur to the president of our country, suffered from a terrible attempt on his life. One day, after he had dropped off the president, killers for hire followed him, assuming that he was the president, and they riddled the car with bullets. Manuel was taken to the hospital on the verge of death. His wife, desperate, called a leader in our ministry asking for prayer. One of Manuel's legs was so badly damaged that the doctors decided it needed to be amputated. His wife made a covenant with God, and, that night, as I ministered in supernatural power, the Holy Spirit placed in my heart that I should send the healing word for Manuel's life. I declared that God was going to create new bone, flesh, arteries, veins, nerve endings, and so forth, in his leg. The next day, the doctors had their surgical tools ready for the amputation, but when they removed the bandages from Manuel's leg, to their surprise, they found he had a completely healthy leg. It even had new skin!"

⌒

Stand Firm on the Truth, Not on Facts

⌒

Faith is based on the truth. As long as you think you have another option or alternative, you will not commit to believe.

When times get hard, some believers compromise the truth. Yet God doesn't have a "plan B" in reserve, because, if He did, He would no longer be sovereign or eternal, and His kingdom would not be unshakable. We must stand firm and believe what God has said. In the midst of a crisis or problem, we can be certain that He never alters His thoughts, plans, or power toward us and toward our purpose, provision, healing, and deliverance. God doesn't change in regard to these things, and neither should we!

If the doctor declares sickness or death over you, do not accept it. Use God's faith and seize your healing. If you accept the doctor's words, you are conforming to the enemy's desire to destroy you. What the doctor is saying is true and is a temporal fact, but it is not God's *truth* for your life. Our inheritance in Christ is kingdom health. Therefore, cancel the influence of those words with the power of God's faith. Use kingdom currency to seize the miracle and say to the doctor, "I don't accept this diagnosis."

When facts change, feelings also change;
but faith is firmly planted on the truth.

Vene Labans of South Africa was diagnosed with HIV six years ago. A couple of days prior to our conference on the supernatural in East London, South Africa, a friend of Vene's invited her to the meetings. She was reluctant but decided to go. On Sunday, I preached on "The Gospel of the Now," saying that, if you believe, you will receive your miracle. Then I made an altar call for those who were HIV-positive or had cancer. Vene approached the altar, willing to use her faith to be healed. One of my ministers declared healing over her, and she felt heat flowing through her body. The following day, she was scheduled to go to the clinic to obtain her monthly medication, but a friend insisted she should be tested, instead, to confirm her healing. So, Vene asked for a new test. To the glory of God, the results were negative!

In one day, Vene's life was completely transformed. Her sickness was temporary; it came to its end when she encountered the power of God. "This conference has completely changed my life; it has given me joy, health, and everything I needed!" she said.

Faith is where the supernatural begins.

If we conform to what the natural world says, we will accept it as being the last word, and it will rule over us. When such thinking becomes established in our hearts, we are not able to receive the supernatural, and we become magnets for sickness, poverty, lack, depression, and pain. We must establish in our hearts the truth that goes beyond all temporal reality. Receive everything that Jesus provided on the cross, right now!

Truth is the only thing that can defy facts because it is the highest level of reality and operates beyond facts.

Journey into Word & Spirit

1. "Faith acts and stands on what God has already predetermined, generating expectation." What do you believe God has predetermined for you?

2. How may you be walking by sight instead of by faith? Repent of this sin and walk forward in God's grace.

Chapter excerpted from Apostle Guillermo Maldonado, *The Kingdom of Power: How to Demonstrate It Here and Now* (New Kensington, PA: Whitaker House, 2013), 216, 220–233, 235–237.

About the Author

Active in ministry for over twenty years, Apostle Guillermo Maldonado is the senior pastor and founder of King Jesus International Ministry, one of the fastest-growing multicultural churches in the United States, in Miami, Florida. Apostle Maldonado has authored over fifty books and manuals. Visit www.kingjesusministry.org for more information.

THE KINGDOM
HEALTH CARE SYSTEM

Cal Pierce

16

THE KINGDOM HEALTH CARE SYSTEM

Cal Pierce

I f sickness is part of the curse we have been redeemed from (Galatians 3:13), then we can live a long life in health. In Genesis 6:3 (NASB) God tells us how long we can live in health.

> *Then the LORD said, "My Spirit shall not strive with man forever, because he also is flesh; nevertheless his days shall be one hundred and twenty years."*

Redemption re-establishes this covenant that God has given us. Science today has discovered that man can live 120 years with proper nutrition, exercise, and kingdom help. The whole man, in spirit, mind and body, can be preserved complete for 120 years (1 Thessalonians 5:23).

Our age does not determine our health. We have this mindset that when we reach 50 years, it's all down-hill from there. When I reached 50, I started receiving mail from senior groups, health insurance companies, rest homes, and cemetery plot sales people. This wasn't encouraging. Now that I am turning 65, I decided to do something about my health.

I was beginning to fit the picture of a deteriorating senior citizen. God gave me a dream that I was to become strong. He showed me how, at any age, with good nutrition and exercise, our bodies will gain new strength. Within five months, I lost 35 pounds, strengthened my body to have energy that I haven't had in 20 years, and every pain and ache has left. I now tell my staff, "I'm not planning to retire for another 50 years." At our conferences, I now teach and impart, not just the message on healing, but also the message on the health we can have after we are healed.

Journey into Word & Spirit

1. Is the Holy Spirit leading you to make any changes to improve your diet? If so, what are they? Some illnesses can be cured or reversed by good nutrition. Dare to believe that God can and will heal you and that He calls you to maintain that healing.

2. What exercises/type of exercise program are you able to do? Remember that faith acts. Develop a program with the help of your physician, and involve a person trainer and/or family member or friend for support. Dare to believe that you can become more mobile and active, despite any ailments you may suffer. Make sure to take note of what you are able to do that you couldn't do before.

3. Spend some time with the Lord and ask Him to give you a vision of yourself walking in perfect health. Keep that vision at the forefront of your prayers and cast out the old, diseased vision of yourself. Without vision, people perish. (See Proverbs 29:18.) Envision what is to come. Dare to believe!

Chapter excerpted from "The Kingdom Health Care System," October 1, 2009, www.healingrooms.com/index.php?page_id=53.

About the Author

Cal Pierce is the founder and director of the International Association of Healing Rooms, based in Spokane, Washington, which provides a place for sick people to come to receive prayer for healing from trained Christian lay-people. Since the first healing room was built in Spokane in 1999, IAHR has opened hundreds of healing rooms around the world. Cal Pierce has written many books, including *Preparing the Way: The Reopening of the John G. Lake Healing Rooms in Spokane, Washington.*

DARE TO BELIEVE, THEN COMMAND

Smith Wigglesworth

17

DARE TO BELIEVE, THEN COMMAND

Smith Wigglesworth

"Verily, verily, I say unto you, he that believeth on me,
the works that I do shall he do also; and greater works than these shall
he do; because I go unto my Father. And whatsoever ye shall ask in my
name, that will I do, that the Father may be glorified in the Son.
If ye shall ask any thing in my name, I will do it."
—John 14:12–14

J esus is speaking here, and the Spirit of God can take these words of His and make them real to us. *"He that believeth on me...greater works than these shall he do."* What a word! Is it true? If you want the truth, where will you get it? *"Thy word is truth"* (John 17:17), Christ said to the Father. When you take up God's Word you get the truth. God is not the author of confusion or error, but He sends forth His light and truth to lead us into His holy habitation, where we receive a revelation of the truth like unto the noon day in all its clearness.

The Word of God works effectually in us as we believe it. It changes us and brings us into new fellowship with the Father, with the Son, and with the Holy Spirit, into a holy communion, into an unwavering faith, into a mighty assurance, and it will make us partakers of the very nature and likeness of God as we receive His great and exceeding precious promises and believe them. *"Faith cometh by hearing, and hearing by the word of God"* (Romans 10:17). Faith is the operative power.

We read that Christ opened the understanding of His disciples, and He will open up our understanding and our hearts and will show us wonderful things that we should never know but for the mighty revelation and enlightenment of the Spirit that He gives to us.

I do not know of any greater words than those found in Romans 4:16, *"Therefore it is of faith, that it might be by grace."* Grace is God's benediction coming right down to you, and when you open the door to Him—that is an act of faith—He does all you want and will fulfill all your desires. *"It is of faith, that it might be by grace"* (Romans 4:16). You open the way for God to work as you believe His Word, and God will come in and supply your every need all along the way.

Our Lord Jesus said to His disciples, and He says to us in this passage in the 14th of John, "You have seen Me work and you know how I work. You shall do the very same things that I am doing, and greater things shall you do, because I am going to the Father, and as you make petition in My name I will work. I will do what you ask, and by this the Father shall be glorified."

Did any one ever work as He did? I do not mean His carpentering. I refer to His work in the hearts of the people. He drew them to Him. They came with their needs, with their sicknesses, with their oppression, and He relieved them all. This royal Visitor, who came from the Father to express His love, talked to men, spent time with them in their homes, found out their every need. He went about doing good and healing all who were oppressed of the devil, and He said to them, and He says to us, "You see what I have been doing, healing the sick, relieving the oppressed, casting out demons. The works that I do shall ye do also." Dare you believe? Will you take up the work that He left and carry it on?

"He that believeth on me"! What is this? What does it mean? How can just believing bring these things to pass? What virtue is there in it? There is virtue in these words because He declares them. If we will receive this word and declare it, the greater works shall be accomplished. This is a positive declaration of His *"He that believeth on me...greater works than these shall he do,"* but unbelief has hindered our progress in the realm of the spiritual.

Put away unbelief. Open your heart to God's grace. Then God will come in and place in you a definite faith. He wants to remove every obstruction that is in the world before you. By His grace He will enable you to be so established in His truth, so strong in the Lord and in the power of His might, that whatever comes across your path to obstruct you, you can arise in divine power and rebuke and destroy it.

It is a matter of definite and clear understanding between us and God. To recognize that Christ has a life force to put into us, changes everything that we dare to *believe* it will change. He that believes that Jesus is the Christ overcomes the world. Because we believe that Jesus is the Christ, the essence of divine life is in us by faith and causes a perfect separation between us and the world. We have no room for sin. It is a joyful thing for us to be doing that which is right. He will cause that abundance of grace to so flow into our hearts that sin shall not have dominion over us. Sin shall not have dominion; nor sickness, nor affliction. *"He that believeth"*—he that dares to believe—he that dares to trust—will see victory over every oppression of the enemy.

A needy creature came to me in a meeting, all withered and wasted. He had no hope. There was absolute death in his eyes. He was so helpless he had to have some one on each side to bear him up. He came to me and said in a whisper, "Can you help me?" Will Jesus answer? *"He that believeth on me, the works that I do shall he do also; and greater works than these."* *"Behold, I give unto you power...over all the power of the enemy"* (Luke 10:19). These are the words of our Lord Jesus. It is not our word but the word of the Lord, and as this word is in us, He can make it like a burning passion in us. We make the Word of God as we believe it our own. We receive the Word and we have the very life of Christ in us. We become supernatural by the power of God. We find this power working through every part of our being.

Now Christ gives us something besides faith. He gives us something to make faith effectual. Whatsoever you desire, if you believe in your heart you shall have. Christ said, *"Have faith in God. For verily I say unto you, that who-soever shall say unto this mountain, Be thou removed, and be thou cast into the sea; and shall not doubt in his heart, but shall believe that those things which he saith shall come to pass; he shall have whatsoever he saith. Therefore I say unto you, What things soever ye desire, when ye pray, believe that ye receive them, and ye shall have them"* (Mark 11:22–24). *Whatsoever he saith!* Dare to say in faith, and it shall be done. These things have been promised by Christ, and He does not lie.

This afflicted man stood before me helpless and withered. He had had cancer in his stomach. The physicians had operated upon him to take away the cancer from the stomach, but complications had arisen with the result that no food could enter the man's stomach. He could not swallow anything. So in order to keep him alive they made a hole in his stomach and put in a tube about nine inches long with a cup at the top, and he was fed with liquid through this tube. For three months he had been just kept alive but was like a skeleton.

What was I to say to him? *"If thou wouldest believe, thou shouldest see the glory of God"* (John 11:40).

Here was the word of Christ, *"He that believeth on me, the works that I do shall he do also; and greater works than these shall he do; because I go unto my Father."* The Word of God is truth. Christ is with the Father and grants us our requests, and makes these things manifest, if we believe. What should I do in the presence of a case like this? *"Believe the Word."* So I believed the Word which says, *"He shall have whatsoever he saith"* (Mark 11:23). I said, "Go home, and have a good supper." He said, "I cannot swallow." "Go home, and have a good supper," I repeated. "On the authority of the Word of God I say it. Christ says that he that believes that these things which he says shall come to pass, he shall have whatsoever he says. So I say, Go home in the name of Jesus, and have a good supper."

He went home. Supper was prepared. Many times he had had food in his mouth but had always been forced to spit it out again. But I dared to believe that he would be able to swallow that night. So that man filled his mouth full as he had done before, and because some one dared to believe God's Word and said to him, "You shall have a good supper in the name of Jesus," when he chewed his food it went down in the normal way into his stomach, and he ate until he was quite satisfied.

He and his family went to bed filled with joy. The next morning when they arose they were filled with the same joy. Life had begun again. Naturally he looked down to see the hole that had been made in his stomach by the physicians. But God knew that he did not want two holes, and so when God opened the normal passage He closed the other hole in his stomach. This is the kind of God we have all the time, a God who knows, a God who acts, and brings things to pass when we believe. Dare to believe, and then dare to speak, and you shall have whatsoever you say if you doubt not.

A woman came to me one night and inquired, "Can I hear again? Is it possible for me to hear again? I have had several operations and the drums of my ears have been taken away." I said, "If God has not forgotten how to make drums for ears, you can hear again." Do you think God has forgotten? What does God forget? He forgets our sins, when we are forgiven, but He has not forgotten how to make drums for ears.

Not long ago the power of God was very much upon a meeting that I was holding. I was telling the people that they could be healed without my going to them. If they would rise up, I would pray, and the Lord would heal. There was a man who put up his hand. I said, "Cannot that man rise?" The folks near him said he could not, and lifted him up. The Lord healed him; the ribs that were broken were knit together again and were healed.

There was such faith in the place that a little girl cried out, "Please, gentleman, come to me." You could not see her, she was so small. The mother said, "My little girl wants you to come." So I went down there to this child, who although fourteen years of age was very small. She said with tears streaming down her face, "Will you pray for me?" I said, "Dare you believe?" She said, "O yes." I prayed and placed my hands on her head in the name of Jesus.

"Mother," she said, "I am being healed. Take these things off—take them all off." The mother loosed straps and bands, and then the child said, "Mother, I am sure I am healed. Take these off." She had straps on her legs and an iron on her foot about 3½ inches deep. She asked her mother to unstrap her. Her mother took off the straps. There were not many people with dry eyes as they saw that girl walk about with legs just as normal as when she was born. God healed her right away. What did it? She had cried, "Please, gentleman, come to me," and her longing was coupled with faith. May the Lord help us to be just like a simple child.

God has hidden these things from the wise and prudent, but He reveals them to babes. There is something in childlike faith in God that makes us dare to believe, and then to act. Whatever there is in your life that is bound, the name of Jesus and the power of that name will break it if you will only believe. Christ says, *"If ye shall ask any thing in my name, I will do it."* God will be glorified in Christ when you receive the overflowing life that comes from Christ in response to your faith.

Dare to believe. Do you think that truth is put into the Word to mock you? Don't you see that God really means that you should live in the world to relieve the oppression of the world? God answers us that we shall be quickened, be molded afresh, that the Word of God shall change everything that needs to be changed, both in us and in others, as we dare to believe and as we command things to be done. *"Whosoever shall say unto this mountain, Be thou removed, and be thou cast into the sea; and shall not doubt in his heart, but shall believe that those things which he saith shall come to pass, **he shall have whatsoever he saith**"* (Mark 11:23).

Journey into Word & Spirit

1. What do you want to ask of the Lord? Write down your specific request and then find a Scripture listed in the following chapter that corresponds with your request. Pray it out loud, declaring the goodness of God.

2. Do you dare you believe? Whether you have been healed or are still waiting to be healed, will you take up the work that Christ has left to you, carrying it on?

Chapter excerpted from "Dare to Believe, Then Command," *Pentecostal Evangel*, March 30, 1940, smithwigglesworth.blogspot.com/search?q=dare+to+believe%2C+then+command.

About the Author

Smith Wigglesworth (1859–1947), known as the Apostle of Faith, had an international evangelistic and healing ministry. A plumber by trade, Wigglesworth had a dramatic life change when, at age forty-eight, he was baptized in the Holy Spirit and anointed with power for preaching and healing. Signs and wonders characterized his ministry. His unquenchable faith inspired thousands to receive salvation, healing, and the filling of the Holy Spirit.

ONE HUNDRED SCRIPTURES
ON HEALING

Compiled by David Emigh

18

ONE HUNDRED SCRIPTURES ON HEALING

Compiled by David Emigh

The following statements are what God has personally said about healing. To the degree you let them flow into your heart, the healing will flow out to your body. Once God's word is allowed to come alive in the heart, it will change the rest of the person. Be patient; a seed takes time to grow, but once it does, it provides fruit for many seasons.

Old Testament

1. *"I am the LORD that healeth thee"* (Exodus 15:26).

2. *"You shall be buried in a good old age"* (Genesis 15:15 RSV).

3. *"Thou shalt come to thy grave in a full age, like as a shock of corn cometh in in his season"* (Job 5:26).

4. *"When I see the blood, I will pass over you, and the plague shall not be upon you to destroy you"* (Exodus 12:13).

5. *"I will take sickness away from the midst of thee....The number of thy days I will fulfil"* (Exodus 23:25–26).

6. "I will not put any of the diseases you are afraid of on you, but I will take all sickness away from you." (See Deuteronomy 7:15.)

7. "It will be well with you, and your days shall be multiplied and prolonged as the days of heaven upon the earth." (See Deuteronomy 11:9, 21.)

8. "I turned the curse into a blessing unto you, because I loved you." (See Deuteronomy 23:5; Nehemiah 13:2.)

9. I have redeemed you from *"every sickness, and every plague"* (Deuteronomy 28:61; see also Galatians 3:13).

10. *"As your days, so shall your strength be"* (Deuteronomy 33:25 NKJV).

11. *"I have found a ransom* [for you]. [Your] *flesh shall be fresher than a child's:* [you] *shall return to the days of* [your] *youth"* (Job 33:24–25).

12. "I have healed you and brought up your soul from the grave; I have kept you alive from going down into the pit." (See Psalm 30:2–3.)

13. "I will give you strength and bless you with peace." (See Psalm 29:11.)

14. "I will preserve you and keep you alive." (See Psalm 41:2.)

15. "I will strengthen you upon the bed of languishing; I will make all your bed in your sickness." (See Psalm 41:3.)

16. "I am the health of your countenance, and your God." (See Psalm 43:5.)

17. *"No plague shall come near your dwelling"* (Psalm 91:10 NHEB).

18. *"I will satisfy* [you] *with long life"* (Psalm 91:16 NHEB).

19. "I heal all your diseases." (See Psalm 103:3.)

20. "I sent My word and healed you and delivered you from your destructions." (See Psalm 107:20.)

21. "You shall not die but live and declare My works." (See Psalm 118:17.)

22. "I heal your broken heart and bind up your wounds." (See Psalm 147:3.)

23. *"The years of your life will be many"* (Proverbs 4:10 NKJV).

24. "Trusting Me brings health to your navel and marrow to your bones." (See Proverbs 3:8.)

25. "My words are life to you, and health/medicine to all your flesh." (See Proverbs 4:22.)

26. "My good report makes your bones fat." (See Proverbs 15:30.)

27. "My pleasant words are sweet to your soul and health to your bones." (See Proverbs 16:24.)

28. "My joy is your strength." (See Nehemiah 8:10.) *"A merry heart does good, like medicine"* (Proverbs 17:22 NKJV).

29. *"The eyes of them that see shall not be dim, and the ears of them that hear shall hearken"* (Isaiah 32:3).

30. *"The eyes of the blind shall be opened, and the ears of the deaf shall be unstopped"* (Isaiah 35:5).

31. *"The tongue of the stammerers shall be ready to speak plainly"* (Isaiah 32:4). *"Then shall...the tongue of the dumb sing"* (Isaiah 35:6).

32. *"Then shall the lame man leap as an hart"* (Isaiah 35:6).

33. "I will recover you and make you to live. I am ready to save you." (See Isaiah 38:16, 20.)

34. "I give power to the faint. I increase strength to them that have no might." (See Isaiah 40:29.)

35. "I will renew your strength. I will strengthen and help you." (See Isaiah 40:31; 41:10.)

36. *"To your old age...and even to gray hairs I will carry you...and will deliver you"* (Isaiah 46:4 NKJV).

37. "I bore your sickness." (See Isaiah 53:4.)

38. "I carried your pains." (See Isaiah 53:4.)

39. "I was put to sickness for you." (See Isaiah 53:10.)

40. "With My stripes you are healed." (See Isaiah 53:5.)

41. "I will heal you." (See Isaiah 57:19.)

42. *"Your light shall break forth like the morning, your health shall spring forth speedily"* (Isaiah 58:8 NKJV).

43. *"'I will restore health to you and heal you of your wounds,' says the LORD"* (Jeremiah 30:17 NKJV).

44. *"Behold, I will bring [you] health and cure, and I will cure [you], and will reveal unto [you] the abundance of peace and truth"* (Jeremiah 33:6).

45. *"I...will bind up that which was broken, and will strengthen that which was sick"* (Ezekiel 34:16).

46. *"Behold, I will cause breath to enter into you, and ye shall live....And [I] shall put my Spirit in you, and ye shall live"* (Ezekiel 37:5, 14).

47. *"Whithersoever the rivers shall come, shall live:...they shall be healed; and every thing shall live whither the river cometh"* (Ezekiel 47:9).

48. *"Seek Me and live"* (Amos 5:4 NKJV; see also verse 6).

49. "I have arisen with healing in My wings [beams]." (See Malachi 4:2.)

New Testament

50. *"I will, be thou clean"* (Matthew 8:3).

51. "I took your infirmities." (See Matthew 8:17.)

52. "I bore your sicknesses." (See Matthew 8:17.)

53. "If you're sick, you need a physician." (See Matthew 9:12.) "I am the Lord your physician." (See Exodus 15:26.)

54. "I am moved with compassion toward the sick, and I heal them." (See Matthew 14:14.)

55. I heal *"all manner of sickness and all manner of disease"* (Matthew 4:23).

56. *"According to your faith be it unto you"* (Matthew 9:29).

57. I give you *"power against unclean spirits, to cast them out, and to heal all manner of sickness and all manner of disease"* (Matthew 10:1; see also Luke 9:1).

58. "I heal them all." (See Matthew 12:15; Hebrews 13:8.)

59. "As many as touch Me are made perfectly whole." (See Matthew 14:36.)

60. "Healing is the children's bread." (See Matthew 15:26.)

61. "I do all things well. I make the deaf hear and the dumb speak." (See Mark 7:37.)

62. *"If you can believe, all things are possible to him who believes"* (Mark 9:23 NKJV; see also Mark 11:23–24).

63. "When hands are laid on you, you shall recover." (See Mark 16:18.)

64. "My anointing heals the brokenhearted, delivers the captives, recovers sight to the blind, and sets at liberty those who are bruised." (See Luke 4:18; Isaiah 10:27; 61:1.)

65. "I heal all those who have need of healing." (See Luke 9:11.)

66. "I have not come to destroy men's lives but to save them." (See Luke 9:56.)

67. *"Behold, I give you the authority...over all the power of the enemy, and nothing shall by any means hurt you"* (Luke 10:19 NKJV).

68. Sickness is satanic bondage, and you ought to be loosed today. (See Luke 13:16; 2 Corinthians 6:2.)

69. "In Me is life." (See John 1:4.)

70. "I give you life." (See John 6:33.) *"I am the bread of life"* (verse 35).

71. *"The words that I speak unto you, they are spirit, and they are life"* (John 6:63).

72. *"I am come that [you] might have life, and that [you] might have it more abundantly"* (John 10:10).

73. *"I am the resurrection, and the life"* (John 11:25).

74. *"If you ask anything in My name, I will do it"* (John 14:14 NKJV).

75. "Faith in My name makes you strong and gives you perfect soundness." (See Acts 3:16.)

76. "I stretch forth My hand to heal." (See Acts 4:30.)

77. "I, Jesus Christ, make you whole." (See Acts 9:34.)

78. "I do good and heal all that are oppressed of the devil." (See Acts 10:38.)

79. "My power causes diseases to depart from you." (See Acts 19:12.)

80. *"The law of the Spirit of life in [Me] has made [you] free from the law of sin and death"* (Romans 8:2 NKJV).

81. "The same Spirit that raised Me from the dead now lives in you, and that Spirit will quicken your mortal body." (See Romans 8:11.)

82. "Your body is a member of Me." (See 1 Corinthians 6:15.)

83. *"Your body is the temple of the Holy Ghost....Glorify* [Me] *in your body"* (1 Corinthians 6:19–20).

84. "If you'll rightly discern My body which was broken for you, and judge yourself, you'll not be judged, and you'll not be weak, sick, or die prematurely." (See 1 Corinthians 11:29–31.)

85. "I have presented gifts of healing to members of My body [the body of Christ]." (See 1 Corinthians 12:9.)

86. "My life may be made manifest in your mortal flesh." (See 2 Corinthians 4:10–11.)

87. "I have delivered you from death; I do deliver you; and if you trust Me, I will yet deliver you." (See 2 Corinthians 1:10.)

88. "I have given you My name and have put all things under your feet." (See Ephesians 1:20–22.)

89. "I want it to be well with you, and I want you to live long on the earth." (See Ephesians 6:3.)

90. "I have delivered you from the authority of darkness." (See Colossians 1:13.)

91. "I will deliver you from every evil work." (See 2 Timothy 4:18.)

92. "I tasted death for you. I destroyed the devil, who had the power of death. I've delivered you who, through fear of death, were subject to bondage." (See Hebrews 2:9, 14–15.)

93. "I wash your body with pure water." (See Hebrews 10:22; Ephesians 5:26.)

94. "Lift up the weak hands and the feeble knees. Don't let that which is lame be turned aside but rather let Me heal it." (See Hebrews 12:12–13.)

95. "Let the elders anoint you and pray for you in My name, and I will raise you up." (See James 5:14–15.)

96. "Pray for one another, and I will heal you." (See James 5:16.)

97. "By My stripes, you were healed." (See 1 Peter 2:24.)

98. "[My] *divine power has given to* [you] *all things that pertain to life and godliness, through the knowledge of* [Me]" (2 Peter 1:3 NKJV).

99. "*Whosoever will, let him* [come and] *take the water of life freely*" (Revelation 22:17).

100. "*Beloved, I wish above all things that* [you may] *prosper and be in health*" (3 John 2).

Chapter taken from http://hopefaithprayer.com/scriptures/100-things-god-said-about-healing-david-emigh/.